MW00778913

Other books by
Denise Carrington-Smith

Outshining Darwin -
Lamark's Brilliant Idea

Engima of Evolution
and the Challenge of Chance

Lord Lucan and Lady Luck -
The murder that never was

Journeyings

Along the path
with
Edward Bach

From Rock Rose to Rock Water

Denise Carrington-Smith

Illustrations
by
Sandra Love

Storixus

First edition published by Abbey Books - 1995
Second edition published by Mossman Print - 2015

Third Edition published 2020 by
Storixus Independent Publishing
Canberra, Australia

www.storixus.com

ISBN 978-0-6483640-5-4 (Paperback Edition)
ISBN 978-0-6483640-6-1 (eBook Edition)

This book is respectfully dedicated
to

DR. ROBERT T. COOPER

physician, the connecting link
between two great healers,
Dr. Samuel Hahnemann
and
Dr. Edward Bach

Acknowledgements

I acknowledge, with thanks, the help and support I have received from my family, my friends, my students and my patients. You have been my teachers and my inspiration. Thank you — each and every one.

A very special thank you to Sandra Love for the beautiful illustrations.

To all others, above and beyond, who have contributed in their own way to bringing this work to fruition — thank you.

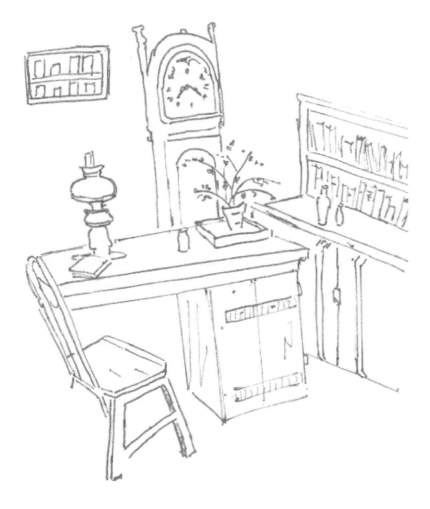

"Thou shalt be missed because thy seat will be empty"

Dr Bach's Study - artist's impression

Foreword

The mind and spirit play a key role in the healing of every human being. Physical techniques are never enough on their own to restore complete health - especially when we are faced with chronic or life-threatening illnesses.

Over the years various forms of counselling and psychotherapy have been evolved to help people make the psychological shift to health. More recently the great value of meditation and hypnotherapy has been realised.

The Bach Flower Essences are also a very useful adjunct in the healing process. They can be used to soothe a distressed person, to act as a catalyst to release inner psychological blocks, to assist in the shifting of difficult emotional states and in the promoting of the desired states.

Dr. Edward Bach was a very sensitive, a very aware and a truly compassionate man - he was a true healer. He gave the world a great gift with his flower essences and with his books inspired by them.

Denise Carrington-Smith's book further expands on Dr. Bach's original insights and adds many useful points gained fron her extensive clinical experience.

This volume deserves to be read by all serious students of Bach Flower Essences.

RALPH BALLARD M.B., B.S., F.A.M.A.S
Cert Manual Medicine
Dip. Homœpathy, Dip. Clinical Hypnosis
Wholistic Medical Practioner

Preface

When teaching the use of the remedies discovered by Dr. Edward Bach, first as Vice-Principal of the Melbourne College of Naturopathy and later as Principal of The Victorian College of Classical Homœopathy, I chose to present the remedies to my students in the order in which they had been given by Dr. Bach in his seminal work, *The Twelve Healers and other Remedies*.

Dr. Bach offered no explanation for the order in which he presented his seven groups, nor for the order in which the remedies appeared within the groups, which was not alphabetical. However, I felt sure there had to be one and soon realized that the remedies did follow on from one another.

I read in Nora Week's biography, *The Medical Discoveries of Edward Bach, Physician*, that Dr. Bach had been working on pairing his thirty-eight remedies, believing the first nineteen he had discovered related in some way to the last, but died after having worked out only a few of the pairings. One day, while going over my notes in preparation for a course of lectures I was to give, the solution dropped, unbidden, into my mind. It was not the first nineteen remedies discovered which paired with the last nineteen, but the first nineteen presented which paired with the last nineteen. It took me but minutes to confirm this truth to myself.

The first remedy is Rock Rose, the remedy for terror, the last Rock Water, the remedy for the person in complete control of themselves and their life. Clearly the one is the partner/antithesis of the other. Likewise, remedy two, Aspen, is partnered by remedy thirty-seven, Beech, and so on, until remedy nineteen, Water Violet, is found to be the partner/antithesis of Impatiens.

Dr. Bach stated that his remedy was Impatiens, the quick thinking, quick acting person who prefers to work alone, but surely Dr. Bach was also Water Violet, the quiet thinking, independent person who spends hours thinking things over, alone, before coming to a conclusion and making a decision to act? His hours of quiet contemplation as he walked the Welsh and English countryside, both as a child and later while actively seeking his remedies, can be no other remedy than Water Violet.

This book is based upon, not only what I learnt from my reading, but also on what I learnt from my students and, more importantly, my patients! Their reaction (or lack thereof!) to the remedies I prescribed, taught me so much. My experience, both as a natural therapist and as a psychologist, taught me that patients frequently present first with one side of their nature uppermost and then with the other. Alternating the paired remedies can be very helpful. I also found it helpful to take note of the two remedies appearing before and after the presenting remedy. My most outstanding results always followed the prescription of a single remedy. However, not all patients responded completely to a single prescription. As one set of symptoms faded, they were often replaced by another. Healing was rather like peeling away the proverbial skins of an onion. That was when an understanding, not only of the before and after remedy, but also of the paired remedy, was invaluable.

Dr. Bach's simple booklet presented remedies to help us as we travel through life, both on our journey through this, our individual life, but also as we, as an individual soul within the greater Soul of humanity, travel the path from our first incarnation to our final perfection.

Denise Carrington-Smith
Mossman
Qld, 4873

October 2015

Preface to Third Edition

In Chapter 4 of this book, I draw attention to Dr,. Bach's obvious interest in the numbers (numerology) — three, four, seven, twelve. Was he also interested in astrology? Eastern philosophy? the chakras?

Eastern philosophy holds that we have seven entergy centres (chakras), five associated with the physical body and two, centred in the cranium, associated with energy (thought). Did the seven goups of remedies relate to the seven chakras? Did the first group, dealing with the most primitive of negative emotions, fear, relate to the base chakra (muladhara), the seventh group to the crown chakra (Sahasrara), manifestion of control, of circumstances and self? Those interested in these things may like to give it consideration.

We know that Dr. Bach believed all living things, including plants, had some degree of consciousness, of awareness. He believed that plants could communicate, mostly between themselves but occasionally with humans. Did he also believe the Earth was a living being? Some people do. They call Mother Earth 'Giai'. Does the Earth have chakras? The Hindoos associated the seven colours of the rainbow with the seven chakras, red being the colour of the base chakra, which could related to Earth's hot, molten interior, on through the green of the vegetation to the blue of the skies. Are their two 'mental' chakras, the purple and the violet of Earth's atmosphere, with its electrical fields and radio waves?

So much to ponder about our beautiful world; so much to appreciate.

Denise Carrington-Smith
Port Douglas.

May 2020.

Contents

Bach Flower Essences

1. Rock Rose	38. Rock Water
2. Mimulus	37. Beech
3. Cherry Plum	36. Vine
4. Aspen	35. Vervain
5. Red Chestnut	34. Chicory
6. Cerato	33. Crab Apple
7. Scleranthus	32. Oak
8. Gentian	31. Willow
9. Gorse	32. Star of Bethlehem
10. Hornbeam	29. Sweet Chestnut
11. Wild Oat	28. Elm
12. Clematis	27. Pine
13. Honeysuckle	26. Larch
14. Wild Rose	25. Holly
15. Olive	24. Walnut
16. White Chestnut	23. Centaury
17. Mustard	22. Agrimony
18. Chestnut Bud	21. Heather
19. Water Violet	20. Impatiens

Chapter One

How it all began

When Charles Dickens wrote his novel, *Oliver Twist*, he became a prime mover in a train of events, the ramifications of which the world is still feeling today. He stirred the social conscience of Victorian Britain by his graphic portrayal of the conditions prevailing in the dreaded workhouses, those refuges to which the destitute turned for help in their time of need. No one was ever turned away; there was food and shelter for any who asked, free of charge, the Spartan conditions ensuring that only those in real need would apply for shelter within those grim walls.

It was a rough and ready Social Security system, through which society provided for its less fortunate members. It had its faults and its critics but served a useful purpose. Nor were the sick forgotten. It was the custom for doctors to charge their patients according to their pockets — the wealthy upper classes paying dearly for the privilege of the doctor's visit, the majority paying a more reasonable fee, while the poor went 'on the panel', receiving their treatment free of charge.

There was one glaring difficulty with this medical system.

Treatment might be free but there was no protection against loss of wages for those too sick to work. Young Edward Bach (1886-1936) growing up in post Dicken's England, watched with great concern workers in his father's brass foundry reporting for duty when obviously sick because they simply could not afford to stay home. This worried the growing boy, as the twin problems of poverty and sickness have worried so many others.

But Bach was not content to dismiss the situation as being too hard for one of his tender years to solve. He turned his attention, not to poverty (the universal, perennial problem which the Great Master said would always be with us) but to sickness and its place in the universal scheme of things. If sickness was the pre-ordained lot of mankind, to be suffered according to the inscrutable Will of God, would the Great Master have devoted so much of his time to healing the sick?

As a young lad, the future Dr. Bach dreamed of finding a simple, safe, effective and economical means of healing, which could be available to all, without the need for the intervention of a physician.

Along with the beasts of the field, we share the instinct to feed when hungry, to drink when thirsty. Yet animals seem to have a better understanding than do we of how to behave and treat themselves in sickness. Dr. Bach felt that within the great scheme of things redressing the imbalance which led to sickness should be as straightforward as redressing the imbalance which resulted in hunger or thirst. He dreamed of the day when he would be able to discover such a system. It was to be many years before the young Dr. Bach came to read the writings of another doctor and healer, Samuel Hahnemann (1755-1843), but, when he did, he instantly recognized a kindred spirit.

Late in the eighteenth century, Dr. Hahnemann had sat through long nights at the bedside of his sick children, his heart crying out for a simple and safe means of restoring their health. His medical training had given him an armament of dangerous poisons with which to fight disease — but at what cost?

"If I", he mused, "an earthly father can long so intensely to restore my little child safely and rapidly to health and happiness, how much more must the Heavenly Father yearn for our healing! Could it be possible that such a loving Divine Father would leave his earthly children without a sure and safe way of overcoming their ills?"

And thus it was that these two great men, Samuel Hahnemann and Edward Bach, separated in time by more than a century yet joined together by one thought, devoted their entire lives to the solving of this sublime problem. Each left to the world a system of healing which was simple, safe, effective and gentle.

The two systems of healing bear both striking similarities and striking differences. Dr. Hahnemann's system of homœopathic remedies is suited to professional use. Although its principle is simple, its practice takes many years of study. The flower remedies discovered by Dr. Bach, now known as the Dr. Bach Flower Essences, are suited to use within the home, being simple in both concept and application. It is to this latter method that this book is dedicated.

Chpater Two

Foundations

The story of Dr. Bach's early years in medical practice, of his work as a bacteriologist, both at University College Hospital and later at the London Homœopathic Hospital, and his subsequent use of the 'sun' method for preparing his herbal remedies, have all been told in the biography written by his long-time friend and co-worker, Nora Weeks (1897—1974).

This book tells of Dr. Bach's growing dissatisfaction with orthodox attitudes towards healing, of his work in developing bacteriological auto-vaccines and of his discovery that optimum response to these auto-vaccines was obtained if a subsequent dose was not administered until the beneficial effects of the former dose had worn off. Dr. Hahnemann, whose work Dr. Bach was to study so closely, had come to the same conclusion with regard to his homœopathic medicines.

Weeks' further tells of Dr. Bach's growing realization during his years as an intern that the crucial factor in the recovery (or otherwise) of many a patient was the patient himself. People with a similarly diagnosed disease, given similar medication, frequently had quite different responses. Dr. Bach came to be able to predict which patients would respond and which would not as he watched different physiological and psychological types react to various treatments.

He became convinced that disease, especially chronic disease, was a crystallization of negative emotions or states of mind. In this understanding also, Dr. Bach later realized that he had but rediscovered a principle outlined over a century before him by the great Dr. Hahnemann.

Dr. Bach carefully studied Hahnemann's work, and at one time incorporated Hahnemann's special method of preparing his remedies into his own bacteriological work. Hahnemann reduced the toxicity of his starting materials by an extensive serial dilution but increased their power by subjecting them to 'succussion' — striking the bottle strongly a number of times against a leather bound book. It is still not understood why this should strengthen the action of the remedy but countless thousands of homœopaths and millions of their patients the world over attest that it does.

In his study of disease, Dr. Bach went further than Dr. Hahnemann in that he claimed that the emotional state was not only the principal but the sole consideration upon which the choice of medication should be based. He, himself, had suffered a severe life-threatening illness. Believing himself to have but a short time to live, he flung himself into his work with all his heart, determined to complete as much as possible before his death. To his surprise he realized that his health had improved.

His work load had not changed but his attitude had. Dr. Bach argued to himself that, if a way could be found to change negative states of mind into positive, healthy states, then it should be possible, not only to slow down, or even prevent, the onset of illness, but it should also be possible to help any already present to ease or lift away.

Dr. Bach came to appreciate the connection between traumas in life and subsequent ill health — a connection being increasingly recognized today, especially with regard to cancer and heart disease. It was not that negative life situations induced disease, *per se*, but rather it was the individual's attitude and reaction to such life situations which brought about subsequent health problems.

A later researcher, Victor Frankl, found that the ability to survive the deprivations of war-time concentration camps depended not so much on physical as on emotional strength. The ability to find meaning in suffering led to less hatred, resentment and thoughts of revenge.

How easy it is to say to someone "Cheer up"- how hard it is to do! Most people are aware of their depression, unhappiness, ill-will, and so on, but trying to cast it aside seems as hard at times as pulling oneself up by the proverbial boot laces. A shallow, temporary state of mind may be overcome by "whistling a happy tune", in much the same way that one may overcome some slight physical indisposition by refusing to allow it to take hold, but, once developed, neither physical nor emotional states of disease so easily yield.

Hahnemann firmly believed that God had placed on the face of the Earth a healing remedy for every disease natural to man, and it was to the plants, minerals and other natural substances that he turned for these remedies. After reading Hahnemann's work, Dr. Bach forsook the bacteriological vaccines he had developed, determined, like Hahnemann, to discover within the realm of Nature the simple remedies he sought to heal mankind.

Hahnemann had already trained as a medical practitioner before coming to realize the need for an improved method of healing. In his early days, Hahnemann attended to his patients' needs in the time-honoured manner, giving chief consideration to their physical symptoms when selecting his treatment and medicine. It was only later that he came to realize the importance of 'mental' symptoms — the emotional and moral state of the patient.

Dr. Bach was different in that he had set out on his medical studies already with the aim of finding a better way. He undertook orthodox studies in order to learn all he could about the system he believed to be inadequate, so that he would know upon what he could build and what he should cast aside. He studied medicine with a questioning mind.

He reached his conclusions regarding the importance of emotions before he broke away from orthodox medicine to seek the alternative of which he had dreamt as a child — that alternative which would be safe, easily available and simple enough for anyone to use.

Chapter Three

Cooper's Contribution

And so it was to the flowers of the field that Dr. Bach turned to find his universal remedies. Of course, herbs have been used for healing purposes throughout recorded history and, no doubt, for many millennium prior, but most frequently the parts of the plant used were the roots, the bark, the leaves or the seeds.

Rarely was the flower used for curative purposes, although chamomile and calendula (marigold) were notable exceptions.

The flower is usually the least toxic part of the plant, although, once again, there are exceptions. The least toxic part of the plant, the flower, has the least physiological effect but the greatest psychological effect.

There is not a human being alive, nor has there ever been, whose heart has not been uplifted by the sight of flowers. In our times of joy and our times of sadness, it is to flowers that we turn. Like the rainbow and the sunset, they speak to our souls. Alas, rainbows and sunsets cannot be relied upon to present themselves exactly at our hour of need! Nor have we yet found a way of capturing their energy and beauty to help heal our hurts. Flowers are easier to obtain — but which flowers? for which need? and how to capture their essence for our use.

Weeks' biography tells of Dr. Bach's hours of meditation, of his quickening psychic abilities which enabled him to select from among a multitude of plants a small number of completely non-toxic flowers, whose high vibrations were of a positive polarity corresponding to, and able to reverse, the thirty-eight negative states of mind to which Dr. Bach believed mankind was subject. Dr. Bach needed a method of potentizing his flower remedies to enhance their action, but the method developed by Hahnemann, which Dr. Bach initially adopted, reversed the energy polarity, essential for the toxic substances utilized in homœopathy but counterproductive for those of positive polarity to which Dr. Bach confined himself.

Dr. Bach utilized the energy from the sun to potentize his early remedies. He insisted on preparing his tinctures immediately the flowers were picked by floating them in a bowl of water placed in the sun beside the mother plant. Later, Dr. Bach was to use heat (simmering) for those of his remedies prepared at times of the year when the sun's strength was insufficient for his purpose.

Another doctor, Robert Cooper (1844—1903), working in London at the turn of the 19th/20th centuries, some thirty years before Dr. Bach, used the same method of preparation, placing the flowers and shoots of growing plants in proof spirit and exposing them to the sun. He called these tinctures 'Arborivital'. An alternative method used by Dr. Cooper was to lower the living branch or stem into the liquid and expose it to sunlight while thus immersed. These tinctures Dr. Cooper called 'Heliosthened'. Dr. Cooper was renowned for his successful treatment of many difficult cases of cancer using these remedies, which he prescribed in 'unit' doses — i.e. one drop at a time.

Although rejected by many mainstream homœopaths, Dr. Cooper had a small band of loyal followers, known as the 'Cooper Club'. One member was Dr. J. H. Clarke, who later became a close friend of Dr. Bach. Dr. Clarke was himself a renowned homœopath, author of a three-volume Materia Medica which is still in great demand today.

In Weeks' biography we read "The evening before he [Dr. Bach] left London, he was greatly encouraged by the words of one physician, Dr. J. H. Clarke, who said to him

> "My lad, forget all you have learnt, forget the past and go ahead. You will find what you are seeking, and when you have found it I will welcome you back and give you my support. I have not long to live, but may I live to see the day of your return, for I know what you find will bring great joy and comfort to those for whom we, at present, can do so little. I shall be prepared to give my work to the flames, and set up instead as a practitioner of the new and better medicine you will find."

Dr. Clarke lived to hear of the finding of the herbal remedies called "The Twelve Healers" and before he died he published the first account of them in his journal, The Homœopathic World.

Dr. Cooper had paid little attention to the mental state of his patients, basing his selection of remedy rather on the organ or tissue involved. His son, Dr. Le Hunt Cooper, continued his work and was a fellow homœopath with Dr. Bach during the latter's time at the London Homœopathic Hospital.

Dr. Bach's uniqueness lay not in the method of preparation, but in the method of selection and application of his remedies.

The similarities in the conclusions reached by Drs. Hahnemann and Bach are quite remarkable. Both taught that disease originated on the non-material plane: in the vital dynamis said Dr. Hahnemann; in negative emotions said Dr. Bach. Neither looked for a primary physiological response to their healing medicines.

Both looked for an adjustment in the inner vibratory level of the patient, to achieve which end only the tiniest amount of physical matter was necessary, to act as a vehicle for the healing energy which would bring about such adjustment to the body or the mind as might be required. Both used extremely small doses of their chosen medicines which, in each case, had been raised to a higher vibratory level by a process of 'potentization'. We see a great unity of thought between these two immortal healers.

In the introduction to his book, The Genius of Homœopathy, Dr. Stuart Close paid tribute to Hahnemann, and other great personalities. His words were written before Dr. Bach's work was published but they apply as much to Dr. Bach as they do to Hahnemann.

> "To each in his own sphere and period, the world comes, and must come, for instruction, inspiration and leadership.
>
> Lesser lights and lesser leaders there must and always will be, to whom, each in his own rank and degree, honour and loyalty are due; but the disciple is never above his master. He only is "The Master" to whom the first great revelation is made and by whom it was first developed and proclaimed; for such epochal men are supremely endowed and specially prepared, usually by many years of seclusion, intense thought and labour. They are raised up at last to do a great work."

Chapter Four

Further Developments

In a paper published in the British Homœopathic Journal during 1920, Dr. Bach made this interesting observation:

> "Individuals having unusual fears, such as a dread of fire, heights, crowds, traffic, have almost invariably an organism of the paratyphoid group bacilli in their gut. The highly strung, nervy person with anxious expression, often with a fixed look, frequently has a bacillus of the proteus group. The patient who at a casual glance appears to be in perfect health and yet has some serious chronic disease often has organisms of the coli mutable group. The folk who bruise and bleed easily generally possess a dysentery type of germ, and so on."

The quotation is of interest, not only because it shows that nine years before embarking upon the final stage of his work, Dr. Bach was already relating mental states to specific bacteria or disease states, but because it illustrates the half-way stage in Dr. Bach's thinking. He commenced by speaking of mental symptoms (fears), but finished by speaking of purely physical symptoms (bruising and bleeding).

In his early bacteriological work, Dr. Bach isolated seven groups of non-lactose fermenting bacteria which he associated with states of disease. He must have been powerfully struck by this number, as a study of Dr. Bach's writings soon makes it evident that numbers held a special significance for him. Of course, this was nothing new. Numbers have played an important part in metaphysical thought since the dawn of recorded history. Such thinking is evident in the Bible, from the seven days of Creation in the book of Genesis to the Seven Churches in the book of Revelation.

Dr. Bach wished to replace his seven groups of bacterial vaccines with seven herbs, as he became more and more convinced that the healing vibrations he was seeking would be found among the beautiful living plants of nature. In 1928 he found the first three, but continued to work on his vaccines for a further two years before abandoning them altogether in favour of his new method. However, he maintained his seven basic groups, replacing the bacilli with seven emotions: peace, hope, joy, faith, certainty, wisdom and love, which Dr. Bach described as "the seven beautiful stages in the healing of disease" (Howard and Ramsell 1990).

Dr. Bach also mentioned twelve positive qualities: love, sympathy, peace, steadfastness, gentleness, strength, understanding, tolerance, wisdom, forgiveness, courage and joy. Only four qualities of the first group appear in the second, and it would seem that Dr. Bach's interest was in presenting seven qualities to represent the seven groups originally represented by the seven bacilli, and twelve qualities to match the twelve healing herbs which he had at that time discovered. He also outlined twelve negative states of mind which he claimed were the true cause of disease.

Another interesting article was published in Homœopathic World in 1930. In this Dr. Bach told of the method he was then using for the preparation of his remedies. After explaining the 'sun' method, he went on to say "about a quarter of the fluid was drawn off at the third, fourth and seventh hours, and about 20 per cent of pure alcohol added to each. This may be used as a third, fourth and seventh potency." Although Dr. Bach later abandoned this concept of different potencies for his remedies, his interest and belief in numerology is plain.

In another article published earlier that same year, Dr. Bach described his preparation of Impatiens, Mimulus and Clematis by the traditional homœopathic method of trituration (grinding) and succussion: "Trituration was done up to the seventh centesimal, after which succussion was adopted." Dr. Bach's decision to triturate to the seventh centesimal potency almost certainly stemmed from metaphysical roots. At the end of this same paper, Dr. Bach stated that the remedies could all be obtained from the third to the twenty-eighth (four times seven) centesimal potencies. Homœopaths traditionally used the 6th and 30th potencies.

Dr. Bach was also interested in astrology. In a letter dated 29th October, 1933, he wrote: "I am being very cautious as regards astrology and that is why one left out the Signs and the months in the first Twelve Healers. This work is decidedly going to assist vastly in the purification and understanding of astrology, but my part seems to be to give general principles whereby people like you who have a more detailed knowledge may discover great truth. That is why I do not wish to be associated with anything dogmatic, until one is sure" (Howard and Ramsell 1990). This letter is illuminating, not only because it shows clearly Dr. Bach's interest in astrology, but because it indicates that Dr. Bach's work formed part of a far larger picture, the final pieces of which are yet to be put in place.

Dr. Bach maintained his seven groups throughout the remainder of his life. His final work, *The Twelve Healers and Other Remedies*, presented the thirty-eight remedies in seven groups, designated, not by seven positive qualities, but by seven negative states.

When Dr. Bach had discovered twelve flower remedies, he published his book under the title The Twelve Healers. He believed he had found the remedies to counter-balance the twelve negative states of mind of which he had at that time spoken: fear, terror, mental torture or worry, indecision, indifference, doubt, over concern, weakness, self-distrust, impatience, over-enthusiasm and pride. As his work developed, he added first a further four, and then another seven, Helpers. (Twelve astrological signs and seven planets?)

During the last year or so of his life, he added a further nineteen remedies, which he believed complemented the action of the first nineteen. Of these, he wrote:

> "The prescription of these new remedies is going to be much more simple than at first appeared, because each of them corresponds to one of the Twelve Healers or Seven Helpers. For example, supposing a case is definitely Clematis and does fairly well but not a complete cure, give the corresponding new remedy further to help the cure. Enclosed is a list of those already worked out; the rest we shall receive in due time."
>
> (Howard and Ramsell 1990)

What happened to the list? Was it ever completed?

Dr. Bach's death did not take him by surprise. He knew that

his contribution was complete and that he would shortly depart. If he had completed the list, one would have expected him to make sure it was adequately recorded before he passed on. Perhaps he abandoned the idea?

The first twelve remedies discovered by Dr. Bach were Impatiens, Mimulus, Clematis, Agrimony, Chicory, Vervain, Scleranthus, Cerato, Water Violet, Gentian and Rock Rose. These were Dr.Bach's "Twelve Healers". The next four remedies discovered were Gorse, Oak, Heather and Rock Water. These Dr. Bach called "The Four Helpers".

The next three added marked a departure from his normal method of discovery inasmuch as Dr. Bach 'knew' what flowers he needed and then obtained them, rather than testing flowers for their possible healing properties. Dr. Bach had to wait several months for the correct season to harvest the Wild Oat and sent directions to colleagues overseas for the harvesting and preparation of Olive and Vine. As more remedies were discovered, Dr. Bach referred to his remedies as "*The Twelve Healers and Other Remedies*".

The above-named remedies constituted the first nineteen, which Dr. Bach believed would be paired with one of the last nineteen, as explained above. Of these nineteen pairings, I believe sixteen do constitute one of the first nineteen remedies discovered, paired with one of the later nineteen. The remaining six are paired with each other: Rock Rose/Rock Water, Scleranthus/Oak and Water Violet/Impatiens.

Are the pairings here suggested correct? And did Dr. Bach know about them before he died? I leave you to judge.

With deep respect for the Master Healer through whom came the revelation of the power of these simple herbal remedies, let us journey along the path outlined by Dr. Bach, and follow the development of the soul from its first descent to its final perfection.

Chapter Five

For those who have fear
(Group One)

Dr. Bach left to us only one small booklet: "The Twelve Healers and Other Remedies" in which he outlined the use of his thirty-eight flower remedies. These he divided into seven groups, each of which will be discussed in the following seven chapters. The remedies were not presented in alphabetical order. No explanation for their order has ever been suggested. I believe there was a plan, an order, although whether Dr. Bach was aware of it or not, I am as yet undecided.

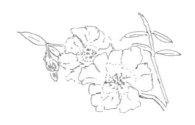

Rock Rose
(Helianthemum nummularium)

The first remedy is Rock Rose. This is a small plant with a yellow flower — not to be confused with *Cistus ladinaferis*, another much larger plant with a pinkish-red flower, also known as Rock Rose, at least in Australia.

This is the remedy originally designated by Dr. Bach 'the rescue remedy', to be used in emergency situations where there is great terror or fright, where there is a feeling "I have to get away". It is a remedy needed in 'here and now' situations, for accidents, trauma, not only for the person who has been hurt but also for the by-standers. It may be that the terror is greater in the witnesses than in the person who has been injured. "In accidents or sudden illness" were the words used by Dr. Bach. This "sudden illness" may be of a physical or an emotional nature, as in grief or shock.

The grief may be for an event which has happened, such as a death, a burglary, a failed business venture or loss of employment (particularly if the event is sudden or unexpected) or a failed examination. It may be for an event which has been forecast, such as following the diagnosis of an incurable disease. Anyone in such a circumstance will be profoundly affected and Rock Rose is the appropriate remedy at this time. Later some other remedy may become indicated as the person and/or their family moves through a progression of emotions.

Rock Rose is also the remedy for extreme phobias. In the presence of the fear stimulus, be it a spider, a thunder storm, a closed space, the person will run if they can. If not, they will be transfixed — frozen with fear. For these people, the remedy may be prescribed on an on-going basis, four drops four times daily, rather than hourly or every few minutes, as is necessary in emergency situations.

Another long-term situation for which Rock Rose may be of service is that of nightmares, or night terrors as they are sometimes called. People suffering from these experiences describe them as incorporating feelings of being transfixed, or frozen, of being unable to escape from whatever form their terror has taken. Some nightmares are inexplicable, others follow terrifying experiences, such as being caught up in a robbery or other assault, or having narrowly escaped some disaster. Natural disasters, such as earthquakes, man-made disasters, such as war, accidents, all may result in an emotional trauma which the mind replays during sleep, with its own unpleasant endings.

I would like to illustrate the use of Rock Rose with a case taken from my own files. It was treated with only the one remedy so the positive reaction cannot be attributed to any other. Dr. Bach did permit the mixing of remedies but every Bach Flower Remedy practitioner with whom I have spoken agrees that the best results are obtained when only one or two remedies are prescribed. Indeed, Dr. Bach suggested two remedies, Wild Oat and Holly, which could be prescribed if too many remedies appeared indicated, showing that he also felt less was better. Too many remedies given at one time seems to subdue their individual properties. I always think of the flower remedies as colours on an artist's palette. The blue and the yellow may be mixed to obtain an attractive green, but add red and the result is somewhat less pleasing. Keep adding colours, and the final result is a nondescript brown. The more added, the more each loses its individual vibration.

One day a young lady in her mid twenties presented at my clinic complaining of panic attacks. While chatting to her, I discovered one of her hobbies had been parachute jumping, which, she assured me, she used to enjoy. "At least," she said, "I think I enjoyed it." Asked to explain further, she told me that she used to parachute with her ex boy-friend. After the relationship ended, she stopped jumping. "If I really enjoyed it," she reasoned, "I would have continued." Further thought elicited the fact that her panic attacks had often occurred on her way to the air field. "In fact, now I come to think of it," she mused, "I believe they started after that time my parachute failed to open." Rock Rose worked wonders!

This brings me to the thought — under what circumstances do we experience the greatest terror? Surely, it is when we are faced with the imminent possibility of death, either our own or that of someone dear to us. If we feel so fearful at the prospect of passing from this plane of existence into the next, what, then, must the soul feel when it is faced with the reality of leaving the heavenly sphere to incarnate down here? Absolute terror! Much work has been done in recent times through hypnotic regression and rebirthing techniques to re-create or relive this early experience and the emotion of terror is described again and again.

This, I feel, is the reason why the first remedy presented by Dr. Bach is Rock Rose. I believe that Dr. Bach has traced the path of the soul, from its earliest descent to its fi nal re-ascent in full perfection. This remedy represents the descent of Spirit into matter, the descent of the group soul of

Mankind as well as of the individual soul into the individual body, one or many times. Many of us must experience this terror at the time of birth. Many will re-experience this emotion as we pass along our way. Indeed, we must experience all the negative states of which Dr. Bach wrote, at some time or another. Almost all of these states or emotions will be experienced by everybody at some time every incarnation, unless that incarnation be very short.

Mimulus

(Mimilus guttatus)

The second remedy is Mimulus, which Dr. Bach tells us is for "Fear of worldly things, illness, pain, accidents, of poverty, dark, of being alone, of misfortune. The fears of everyday life." Dr. Bach then gives a little personality picture: "These people quietly and secretly bear their dread; they do not freely speak of it to others."

As we work through the remedies, we will find that a number of them have personality pictures. These indications are for people who manifest the particular qualities or emotions prominently in their life, but every one of us may experience these emotions at some time and will benefit from the remedy without necessarily fitting the personality picture.

Dr. Bach spoke of this remedy being for children. So many children have fears of everyday things — of going to school, of not measuring up to expectations, especially when they are not even sure of the standard against which they are being measured, of that adult world 'out there', the rules of which they might unwittingly transgress. The child that cries, that does not want to go to kindergarten or school, is afraid of joining in the play activities of his/her peer group, the child who bed-wets, all these may respond well to a course of Mimulus.

Mimulus is also the remedy for minor phobias, not the extreme terror or panic of which we spoke with Rock Rose, but the phobia that can be controlled by an effort of the will. In these cases, while the person may well walk up several flights of stairs rather than take the lift, they can ride in the elevator if they have to. The phobia is not crippling their life. Another common fear is that of public speaking. Very few people with an extreme phobia regarding speaking in public will volunteer to do so in the first place, but the Mimulus people may well agree, only to regret their rashness as the time draws near.

There are so many Mimulus situations — fear of an upcoming interview, of starting a new job, of taking one's driving test, fear of illness, fear of dying.

Fear of death can be very acute in young people, especially teenagers who are coming to terms with their own mortality in a way the very young child does not. Some elderly people are afraid of dying, or of being left behind after their partner dies, although they may not talk about it. As Dr. Bach said, "They may quietly and secretly bear their dread". However, do not make the mistake of assuming that all elderly people fear death. When a life draws towards a natural completion, there may be little or no fear. As we long for the blessing of sleep at the end of a busy day, so may the elderly yearn for the blessing of the Great Sleep at the end of a full life.

Although Mimulus is very good for children, it is by no means needed by them alone. One could say that it is of use in any situation in which an adult is feeling like "the child within", whenever a person feels vulnerable, when they would like someone to hold their hand, no matter how young or old they may be.

And how does Mimulus fit into the greater scheme? We left our incarnating soul in its Rock Rose state of terror. Now it has arrived. No wonder it experiences "fear of worldly things" as it evaluates its position and surveys its alien surroundings. How fearful and forsaken must it feel; no wonder the baby feels so much like crying!

Mimulus — for the fear of going forth into the world of experience.

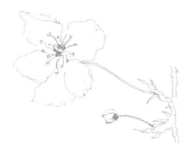

Cherry Plum
(Prunus cerasifera)

In England, there are a number of flowering trees (apple, almond, plum, cherry, among others) which burst into bloom as the winter frosts and snows recede and the sun shines out once more from the clear blue sky.

A few brave plants herald the approach of spring, (the snow drop, the crocus) — then suddenly the equinox is passed, plants and tress burst forth into an incredible display of vibrant blossoms. Spring has come! One can feel the joy in the air, see the spring return to peoples' step. It is hard to be downcast on such a day. Something deep within the heart warms with the upward surging of Life's energy.

From among this group of flowering trees, Dr. Bach found Cherry Plum to be the remedy for a very particular type of fear. The fear corresponding to Cherry Plum is more profound than that of either Rock Rose or Mimulus because it comes from deep within the self.

While all souls are subject to the Rock Rose fear when a traumatic situation occurs, once the situation has passed, equilibrium can be re-established. There may be fear of suffering, a feeling of the situation being out of control, but there is no aggressive or destructive impulse, other than the minimum which may be necessary to escape from an intolerable situation.

The fear of Cherry Plum is different and far more terrible because it is the fear of losing control of the self, of harming self or others. Of all the fears to which mankind is subject, this is the deepest and most destructive. Dr. Bach's description is brief, but within it he encompasses much.

"Fear of the mind being over-strained." This is its first manifestation. It is not a physical over-straining or exhaustion, but a mental one. One such situation with which many people will be familiar is that of the new mother, exhausted to the point of distraction by the demands of her newborn child. No doubt she feels physically drained by the never-ending calls made upon her by her increased family unit. So often this state is observed in first-time mothers, while those with larger families (and, presumably, a heavier work load) cope with an additional infant's demands with less trauma, showing that this is truly an emotional, not merely a physical, state. Other examples are that of a student approaching examination time or of a care-giver coping day after day with a difficult relative/patient.

Whereas Rock Rose is mostly needed in short-term emergency situations, Cherry Plum is indicated more frequently for the results of long-term over-strain. The important indication here is that Dr. Bach included this remedy among those for fear. Exhaustion, whether physical or emotional, is not alone sufficient. There has to be that fear of losing control, "I can't cope any more". If pressed, the person will say, "I'm afraid I will hurt/kill my child/spouse/self". As Dr. Bach has expressed it, "Fear of doing fearful and dreadful things, not wished and known wrong, yet there comes the thought and impulse to do them".

Cherry Plum may be the remedy required for that stage of life known as "the terrible two's", when some toddlers throw temper tantrums. It will only be the appropriate remedy if the tantrums are the result of the child feeling pushed to the limit — not if they are the result of naughtiness or willfulness. Imagine for a moment what it would be like to visit a foreign country, alone, unable to communicate except for a few words supplemented by simple sign language. This must be how a two year old feels at times. Added to this, they are becoming increasingly aware of how practical things, such as tying shoe laces, ought to be accomplished, but their tiny fingers will not co-operate! Just as they are engrossed in some activity, along comes Mother with "into the car, dear, it's time to go to the shops", or, worse still, "It's time for bed". No wonder at times children feel they cannot stand it any more and express their feelings in the only way known to them.

"Things not wished for, known to be wrong, yet there comes the thought and impulse to do them" — this phrase opens up another area of possible use for this remedy, one that I have never had the opportunity to test in practice. Could it be of service for those unfortunate individuals who suffer impulses at times to commit crimes of violence, frequently, but not necessarily, of a sexual nature? We are told these people speak of the thought which implants itself into their mind, which grows more and more insistent, until finally it can be resisted no longer and the deed is done.

If undiscovered, they live in fear of the return of the unwanted impulse. Others are more fortunate in that they never act out their impulses, but the strain of living with unwanted (degrading) thoughts, which enter and dominate their minds, despite their best endeavours, is immense. In a similar situation are those people who hear voices. Some people contemplate suicide as the only way of escape and this is definitely an idea "known to be wrong" yet there comes the thought and impulse to carry it out.

Intense pain, especially if prolonged, can drive people to a state in which they feel they will go mad. The sufferer may even use the phrase "I cannot stand it any more". They are crying out for the blessed relief that Cherry Plum may bring. Remember Cherry Plum in child birth, for injuries, burns, even eczema when the itching drives the patient to distraction.

One further thought — remember this remedy for certain stages of grief. The loss of a loved one can lead to just such a state of over-strain of the mind and of the emotions, the bereaved may even contemplate suicide because they feel they cannot face life without their beloved.

Cherry Plum represents the stage at which an important decision must be taken by the incarnated soul — will it stay and battle the negative forces, which it is now aware reside within itself, not merely in external circumstances or surroundings (Mimulus)? It is not so much "To be, or not to be" as "To stay, or not to stay" that is the question. All souls are faced with this decision many times during the course of their evolution and when the state of anguish is present, Cherry Plum will help uplift the tormented spirit, to enable it to carry on.

One may wonder why Cherry Plum does not follow Rock Rose in Dr. Bach's scheme — they are both remedies for such strong emotions. Why was Mimulus inserted between them? Is it that the Cherry Plum state is a more developed one than that of Mimulus? Only as the developing soul becomes aware of its responsibilities and capabilities for good and evil can this state be experienced.

One could say that this remedy marks the Great Divide between mankind and the animal kingdom. An animal may experience Rock Rose terror or Mimulus fear, but only a human has a sufficiently developed sense of right and wrong, of good and evil, to be driven to a Cherry Plum state. The animal and the human infant act from instinct or desire, untroubled by questions of conscience. Fear of loss of control, of doing that which is known to be wrong, implies that some measure of control, and a knowledge of good and evil, has been attained.

Dr. Bach left the clue to the significance of this remedy in the two words "known wrong".

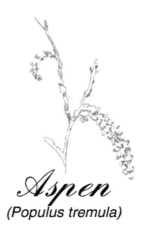

Aspen
(Populus tremula)

Mimulus, we recall, was the remedy for known fears, for fears of worldly things. Aspen is the remedy for fear of unknown things, other worldly things, vague, unknown fears for which there can be given no known explanation, no reason, fears that cannot be expressed in a tangible way.

Said Dr. Bach "These vague, unexplainable fears may haunt by night or day. Sufferers are often afraid to tell their troubles to others", because they cannot explain them, do not understand them themselves, and do not expect the understanding of others.

The Aspen state is one of awareness of realms other than the material. At times the soul senses, but does not understand, that of which it is aware. In endeavouring once again to make contact with the Higher Self, it fi nds that its sensitive antennæ are also tuning in to other unwanted vibrations. Although not all may be harmful, the soul fears that which it does not understand. The soul is aware now of the universality of good and evil, of its existence, not only externally on this plane (Mimulus), not only within the self (Cherry Plum), but on all levels of consciousness.

Although the words used by Dr. Bach to distinguish between

the two remedies, Mimulus and Aspen, appear simple, the choice between them is anything but simple in practice. There are many instances in which an apparently 'known' fear or fear of something worldly, may also be interpreted as an 'unknown' or unreasonable fear. Fear of heights, fear of thunderstorms, fear of the flying, fear of death. All these tangible fears may be Mimulus in one person and Aspen in another. If the fear develops as the result of some traumatic event, then Mimulus may be the most appropriate remedy. If there is no explanation for the fear, or the fear is greatly in excess of that considered 'normal' (whatever that might be!) then Aspen may be more suitable. For example, some people have an unreasonable fear of developing cancer. This fear may haunt them for years, despite negative tests.

On first consideration, this may appear a 'known' or 'worldly' fear, but inasmuch as it is unfounded, or unrealistic, Aspen may be more appropriate.

In choosing between these two remedies, it may be of help to consider the nature of the Aspen tree itself. Its leaves are never still. They quiver and tremble in response to the slightest current of air, even those of which no other plant or person seems to be aware.

The Aspen person might be likened to a spider crouched in the centre of its web, which vibrates from the slightest touch against one of its strands of thread, which it, itself, has woven for its own use. Friend or foe? Predator or prey? Is investigating worth the risk of being devoured? Eventually the soul must learn to face up to the challenges of existence. Until it does, it cannot truly develop its humanity. The paradox of the Aspen state lies in that increasing awareness of other realms of consciousness, of the non-material, brings with it an increasing awareness of the role of mankind in the great drama of Life to be played out upon this physical plane.

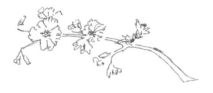

Red Chestnut

(Æsculus carnea)

The cosmic drama has a large cast! The soul in the Red Chestnut stage has become aware of its fellow actors, of how dependent he/she is upon them, and how dependent they are upon him/her.

This is the remedy for those who worry more about others than they do about themselves. Their tranquility is ruined by persistent worrying thoughts about possible dangers or accidents which may threaten their loved ones, when these people are not under their immediate loving and watchful eye.

An infant's fi rst need is for companionship. All babies must go through a Red Chestnut stage because disappearance of their mother, through death or desertion, would mean death to them. Many an adult manifests over-concern for their off-spring because they, themselves, were deprived of emotional support when young. A feeling of being truly loved, appreciated and cared about begets the feeling of confidence as can nothing else. We long to be cared about — and we long to care about others, especially others close to us by reason of ties of family or friendship.

Those manifesting the Red Chestnut state may be blissfully

unaware that the concern they feel is anything other than beneficial for the hapless recipient of their feelings. Others do know and describe themselves as 'worriers'. The recipient is very aware of the true state of affairs. They feel oppressed, for the state of Red Chestnut is that which corresponds to the selfish fear "What will I do if anything happens to my family, my spouse, my care-giver, my friend, my child?" It is the fear of being deserted.

Many children become as over-protective of their parents as their parents are of them. This was beautifully expressed by A. A. Milne in his well-known poem in which Christopher Robin firmly tells his mother .

> "You-mustn't-go-down-to-the-end-of-the-town-if-you-don't-go-down-with-ME!"

Describing Red Chestnut, Dr. Bach said it was "For those who find it difficult not to be anxious for other people. Often they have ceased to worry about themselves, but for those of whom they are fond they may suffer much, frequently anticipating some unfortunate thing may happen to them." We see why this remedy is the last given in the Fear section.

These people have ceased to worry about themselves. This is definitely progress when compared with the Mimulus or Aspen state. It is indeed the state of that unselfish love of which the Great Master spoke when he said "Greater love hath no man than this, that he lay down his life for his friend."

But there is a long developmental road to be trod between the first glimpse of this state and its final perfect manifestation. Then, concern is for the good of the other soul alone. Perfect love overcomes all fear. The purpose of the flower remedies is not to eliminate an emotional state, but to transmute it, bringing it to its most perfect level of expression. Lest we should have too poor an opinion of ourselves, let us remember that the first reaction of most of us, on seeing another person in distress, is to help. Complete strangers will plunge into the water to save another from drowning, brave flames to rescue another from fire. Mankind in essence is heroic and unselfish. It is true that there are times when our baser instincts surface, but natural disasters, such as earthquakes and bushfires, show us that our first instinct is to help. Only on the second or third day after the disaster does the selfish side come to the fore in some people and looting commence.

It may be of benefit to remind ourselves of the circumstances under which Dr. Bach was brought to a realization of the need for this remedy. He suffered a wound from an axe, which invoked instant concern in his companions. He felt this concern, not as a positive, uplifting loving force, but as a wall of fear which impeded, rather than helped, his recovery. There can, I am sure, be no doubt of the genuine love which his companions felt towards him, but, at that instant, their primary emotion was fear, which was felt by him as a negative influence. This negative influence is often referred to as 'smother love'.

How truly did the Buddha speak when he told us to follow the 'Middle Path'. At times it seems less like a path than a tight rope! First, we need to learn to care for our fellow travellers, especially those with whom we share close family ties, then we need to learn to let them go, to emulate the bird who tips its fledgling out of the nest. We all must learn to spread our wings, to answer the challenges of life, to strive to overcome. The wise parent or friend knows when to encourage and when to refrain. How hard it is!

While a Red Chestnut state may manifest at any time, there are four stages of life when it is likely to be prominent. The first is that of infancy, the second that of the teenager (or older person) in love, the third is the parent and the last is the elderly person who lives in fear that their partner will die before them. They wonder how they will face life alone.

This remedy helps us to adjust the rightful concern we feel for our fellow travellers, removing the fear and allowing loving care to manifest unimpeded.

Of the seven beautiful soul healing qualities which Dr. Bach listed, I believe Faith to be the antithesis of Fear. Fear holds us back from achieving so much. It is at the base of so many problems. When fear is replaced by faith, our potential becomes unlimited.

Chapter Six

For those who suffer uncertainty
(Group Two)

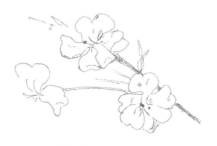

Cerato
(Ceratostigma willmottianum)

While the soul in the Red Chestnut state is over protective and more than willing to give help and advice to family and friends, the Cerato soul manifests the opposite state. These people are the willing recipients of advice and help, so much so that they fail to develop confidence in themselves and their own decisions. "Those who have not sufficient confidence in themselves and their own decisions. They constantly seek advice from others, and are often misguided."

The Cerato person relies too much on the advice and support of others. Of course, it is right and proper that we should listen to the wise counsel of our companions, but, in the final analysis, any decision taken is ours, and ours alone.

In our consideration of Red Chestnut, we spoke of the feeling of confidence which is generated when we know we can rely on the loving support of another human being, of how a Red Chestnut parent is essential for the healthy development of the tiny infant, and of how the infant, also, may experience a Red Chestnut fear when it is separated from its parents or care-giver. Cerato equates to that stage of life when the infant has overcome its fear of being deserted. It no longer suffers a state of fear when its parent leaves for a short time.

Now it needs to learn so much and does so by the continual asking of questions and by the copying of other peoples' words and actions. For this stage of its development, this is useful and constructive behavior. However, there comes a time when it must be left behind. The child needs to become its own person, to take responsibility for its own thoughts and actions.

Whilst most people make this transition satisfactorily, there are some who grow into adult life lacking confidence in themselves. They may be quite intelligent and competent, but feel the need for direction or confirmation from someone else. Such people will feel more comfortable working in a position which has a clearly defined job specification, often in a larger organization with a goodly number of fellow employees who may be consulted on various matters as the Cerato person feels the need.

The professional sales person soon learns to manipulate these unfortunate souls, who may well commit themselves to the purchase of some item they cannot afford, do not want or which they do not like, through the persuasiveness of their arguments.

The sad thing is that Cerato usually knows in their heart of hearts the correct thing to do. After following another person's poor advice, they may say, "What made me do that? I knew I should not." The Cerato person needs to listen to their own inner voice and to learn to trust its guidance.

After infancy, when a Cerato stage is needful, the next developmental stage at which Cerato is likely to dominate is the teenage years. These young people are renowned for their desire to be part of the latest trend, to dress, to speak, to behave, in the manner of their peers.

A further state which is typically Cerato is that of falling in love. At this time, one may put aside one's own decisions and choices in favour of those of the loved one out of a misguided concept of the expression of love. It is a difficult time, because compromise is essential but there should be a giving and a taking. If one partner is manifesting strong Cerato traits, the other may make unsuitable recommendations regarding courses of action. Indeed, it is possible that an unwise marriage may be entered into because of the inability of one person to make a wise decision. The same may be true of business partnerships.

Elderly people may revert to a Cerato state and allow other people to order their affairs in a manner which is not truly to their benefit.

Another manifestation of this state of mind is shown in disciples of a strong leader, be that leader religious, political or from any other domain.

Strong leaders give clear and direct commands or

guidelines and Cerato people feel safe in such an environment. Leaders need their Cerato supporters (they are the ones who do all the hard work!) and so this state, even in an adult, can be beneficial to mankind in general, provided that the leader whom they follow is working for the benefit of mankind and not their own aggrandizement. Thinking back to Red Chestnut, we can imagine the state of fear such followers would endure if their idol's welfare was threatened in any way!

At times, it may be beneficial for the Cerato person to receive strong guidance — they may make worse decisions left to their own devices — but with the help of Cerato they may learn to detach, to stand on their own feet.

An extension of this reliance on the advice or opinion of those perceived to be strong, wise, or even infallible, is that of the person who places his/her trust in psychic readings. While guidance from this source may be invaluable, it is not beneficial to our development to become over-reliant on this advice, any more than on that of any other.

On the physical level, Cerato should be considered as a possible remedy for a patient whose ailments are constantly changing — one day a headache, another day indigestion, another day some other ache or pain. It is as if even their ailments cannot make up their minds.

A further characteristic which is often shown by Cerato is that of having many interests or hobbies. They may change from one to another (often following the forming of new friendships) or they may try to juggle them all within their time schedule. It is not that having a wide range of interests is in itself a bad thing — it is simply that this may serve as a guide to the need for this remedy in some people.

While Cerato serves as a 'type' remedy for those people who exhibit this trait strongly in their day to day lives, every one of us can pass through a temporary Cerato state at times. These are usually times of stress, whether pleasurable or not, such as getting married, having a baby, changing jobs, going overseas, deciding whether or not to have an operation — when others are more than happy to enlighten us with the benefit of their advice and experience, if we are willing to listen.

Enjoy their recommendations and reminiscences, but make your own decision!

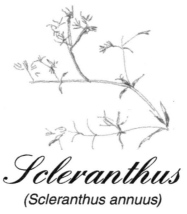

Scleranthus
(Scleranthus annuus)

It is said that the growth of each new baby sees mankind retrace the steps of its physical development over the æons from the single cell to the completed child. With our emotional development, too, the behavior of the infant gradually changes as it grows from self-centred to social behavior of a standard which has allowed civilization to take place. It is believed that a similar retracing also takes place in our spiritual development.

And so it is on our hypothetical journey through life with the Bach remedies. We follow the growth of our soul and see that it has now passed through the state of dependency typified by Cerato. It has reached the stage of its development when it is both capable of, and prepared to make, its own decisions. Now, it is not so much "To be, or not to be?" as "To do, or not to do?" - and what to do — that is the question. This is the big dilemma facing Scleranthus.

"Those who suffer much from being unable to decide between two things, first one seeming right, then the other. They are usually quiet people, and bear their difficulty alone, as they are not inclined to discuss it with others."

The soul is now taking responsibility for its own decisions.

The Scleranthus people have recognized the need to fight their own battles, to make their own decisions, and not to rely on the superficial evaluations of other people, however well meant. This is not to say that Scleranthus people will never benefit from wise counsel. They may well decide to confide in a close friend, or some other person whose opinion they respect, but, after listening, they will consider well that which has been said and make their own decision. While undergoing this, they may suffer much, and Scleranthus is the remedy to help them at this time.

It should be remembered that the more obvious the solution appears to be to other people, the more difficult and deep-seated is the problem. For example, if a woman is being ill-treated by her husband, the most obvious solution might appear to be for her to leave him. If she hesitates to do this, one has to ask "Why?" It may take a long time in counseling before all the issues are explored and brought to some state of resolution. Scleranthus may help to clarify these issues and to bring a sense of certainty about the right course of action.

Dr. Bach said "first one thing seeming right, then the other". He did not say "better" but "right", indicating to us that one of the greatest battles to be fought by the person in the Scleranthus state is that of choosing the right path. At some point, the soul must choose which Path it wishes to follow, that of Darkness or that of Light. Whichever is chosen, that Path is not always followed, either for good or for evil. 'Bad' people do good things and 'good' people do bad things. The soul may wish to change direction and sometimes the choices we face, between the 'easy' way, the way with the most immediate benefit, may not be the 'right' way.

The choices we are called upon to make may not be 'life and death' choices; most choices are far more mundane but, nevertheless, they shape our soul and our destiny. We face many decisions which will either progress us further along the path mapped out for us or will cause us to deviate from it. Happily, wrong decisions are not final within the greater scheme of things. The chance, the lesson, will be re-presented but all of us desire to make the best decision possible on each occasion. At times, it seems very hard. It may be that the more we ponder, the less clear the answer seems. Unlike the Cerato person, Scleranthus does not seek advice from others, but struggles to resolve its own dilemma.

Major decisions must be faced by all teenagers as they consider their future life's work. At school, they must select subjects, they must choose their ongoing training, if any. They must choose between boy/girl friends and, most importantly of all, they must choose their life partner, if any.

Adolescence itself is a Scleranthus state. At birth there is very little difference between a male child and a female child in its relation to life. Until puberty, differences remain comparatively minor, and many which do exist are socially induced. But at puberty a clear decision is made to be male or female. In most cases, this is a decision not within the control of the soul at that time (the decision having been made before incarnating) but some do experience indecision even in this respect. Puberty is the great time of differentiation; it marks the fork in the road.

Scleranthus represents a state of imbalance, either physical or emotional. Its physical manifestation may be in ailments of the body which fluctuate, alternate or move about. This latter indication is similar to that found under Cerato because the two states may not be entirely separated. The Scleranthus state is more an alternation of definite symptoms while Cerato tends to an erratic confusion of symptoms.

The Scleranthus person may stand or sit with the head to one side or with the body in an unbalanced position. Emotionally, the Scleranthus person may exhibit mood swings, being up one day and down the next, especially during their times of doubt.

A state of total indecision may result in no action at all — remember Scleranthus for boredom. This is not quite the same condition as the apathy of Wild Rose, of which we will speak later. The Scleranthus person would be quite willing to participate in some activity if they could decide what to do.

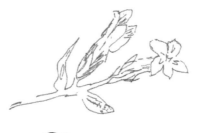

Gentian
(Gentian Amarella)

How pleasing it would be if we could move straight ahead with our Scleranthus decisions made, to fulfill our mission or purpose in life, but, alas, it is seldom so easy. Nothing worthwhile, we are told, is ever easily accomplished. Rarely is anything worthwhile accomplished without setbacks, hindrances or delays, and these often bring with them states of doubt — did I make the correct decision after all? If this is the right path, why are things not going more smoothly?

Dr. Bach tells us that Gentian is the remedy for those who are easily discouraged and, indeed, some people do seem to be more readily disheartened than others. But every cloud has a silver lining and those who tend to be easily discouraged are often those who quickly cheer up again when circumstances improve. Like Scleranthus before them, they may be subject to mood swings, up one minute and down the next.

Some people retain the ability to bounce back throughout life, but others increasingly retain hurts and disappointments and find it harder to be cheerful. This may develop into a state of depression, for which another remedy is needed. Positive examples of Gentian states may be seen in young children, who quickly forgive and forget. Children have short memories for all things, good and bad. The two-edged sword of life dictates that as we collect and retain memories, we will find it harder to forget the bad at the same time that we receive the blessing of recalling the good.

None of us passes through life without feeling disheartened at some stage about something, be it our work, our health, our family, our finances. Those who become discouraged easily when things do not go according to plan may need to take Gentian for some weeks or months as their 'type' remedy. For others, it may be a more unusual situation and they may need Gentian for only a short time, to help them in a particular state of adversity. It matters not — Gentian will help.

Sometimes people in a Gentian state will describe themselves as 'depressed'. This is not the clinical state of depression which is better covered by either Gorse or Mustard. The Gentian state is one of reaction to negative life events, which may be experienced at any time. Children may become discouraged if they do not perform well at school, especially if they fail an examination, and this may have a long-term effect on their self-perception, if not corrected. Whether it will help them perform better, or merely be less concerned about their poor results, time will tell! Even Gentian cannot replace a mediocre brain with that of a genius!

To help clarify the difference between depression and the discouragement or doubt of Gentian, consider the situation of failing an examination, a job interview, or even the breaking up of a friendship. For a while, one may feel disheartened, possibly for a few hours or a few days, but then recover one's cheerfulness, realizing that life holds other opportunities. If the state continues for longer than this, then it may be becoming a true depression and need a different remedy.

The purpose of Gentian is not to allow us to pass through life totally free from any hindrances. It is there to help us achieve the maximum potential from any situation, to allow the negative to be released and the realization to be reached that the past situation was merely a stepping stone to something else, to help us re-assess and move forward. The Bach remedies are not intended to take away our pains and lessons, but to enable us to receive the maximum benefit from life's experiences whatever they may be.

There are three key note indications for Gentian. The first is that the person is able to say about what it is they feel discouraged — there is a known cause of their disheartenment. The second is that there is doubt — doubt about their own abilities, doubt about the eventual outcome of the situation or treatment. The third is that the state is temporary. Two of the three Gentian characteristics are to be found also in Gorse; there is a known cause for their discouragement and there is doubt. The third characteristic has changed from 'temporary' to 'long term'.

Gorse
(Ulex europæus)

When considering Gentian, I spoke of how the young child or person seems better able to throw off life's setbacks. They have greater resilience. Over the years it would seem that repeated hindrances and disappointments have the effect of knocking some of the stuffing out of us.

It used to be said that children pre-puberty do not suffer from depression. This is now debated, but it is generally acknowledged that the capacity to experience depression increases as we grow older. The young child is more pliable, is able to form new friendships, to adjust to new situations, far more easily than the adult. With the ability to retain comes the inability to let go. And with the inability to let go of the past, 'to go with the flow', comes the ability to enter into a state of depression.

This may be the result of many small set-backs or of one

major event, such as a death, diagnosis of an incurable condition, the loss of a limb or a faculty such as sight, a family break-up, a severe financial loss, possibly from failure of a business, loss of employment or betrayal by a friend. Gorse is the remedy to help lift such depression and despondency.

Gorse may also be of service in homesickness, whether the homesickness be temporary while staying away from home, or more permanent as the result of relocation to another locality, or loss of home through fire, flood, earthquake, war, or other suffering.

These circumstances, and many others, may result, not merely in discouragement, but in very great hopelessness. Dr. Bach tells us that the Gorse person has given up the belief that more can be done for them. As a doctor, he spoke in terms of disease, but it is not only as a result of physical disease that we may feel hopelessness. Long term disease is a major cause of depression, both for the sufferer and their care givers. Dr. Bach goes on to say that under persuasion or to please others, these people may try different treatments, at the same time assuring those around them that there is so little hope of relief. Even agreeing to see another therapist (or applying for yet another job) to please another person, is, in itself, a sign of giving up. They cannot argue any more and comply for the sake of peace.

Doubt here is felt more as doubt about the possibility of changing external circumstances than a doubt about oneself.

One must be sensible. There is such a thing as an incurable disease or situation. Some diseases are incurable in the long term; the patient may have years to live in that state. Others are more quickly terminal. Whatever the case, one has to come to terms with the situation. Often it is the parents, spouse, or other relatives who suffer more depression than the person afflicted. The sufferers themselves may display an amazing resilience

We are fortunate in this day of mass media so often to be able to share the story of some brave individual who has overcome adversity and, in so doing, has opened up another vista upon life. This is the role of Gorse in incurable disease, or other unalterable conditions, to help us realize that so long as we are alive (and conscious) there is always something that can be accomplished.

Until death intervenes, one has to carry on, one way or another. Which way is up to us. The Gorse state is one in which death does present as an option to be considered. This suicidal state differs from that of Cherry Plum in that death is welcomed. With Cherry Plum, death is feared.

None of Dr. Bach's thirty-eight remedies is specifically for grief, for grief manifests in many forms, but depression frequently follows the death of a loved one, especially if that death be sudden or unexpected. There is no age limit. The elderly can be as grief-stricken and depressed following the death of their partner as can a younger person for a parent, sibling, child or mate. All may grieve for a friend.

For the hysterical stage of grief, Cherry Plum would be more appropriate.

For guilt, bitterness, there are other remedies.

"So little hope"- how these words pull at the heart-strings! This remedy brings a ray of sunshine to help dispel the gloom.

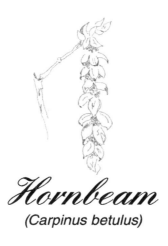

Hornbeam
(Carpinus betulus)

As a child I was taught when stung by a stinging nettle to look for the dock which was sure to be growing nearby, for wherever is the problem, there also will be the remedy.

So it is with these remedies. Following the depression of Gorse comes the turning-point remedy of Hornbeam. "For those who feel they have not sufficient strength, mentally or physically, to carry the burden life placed upon them." It is the pick-me-up remedy.

It will be remembered that our study of Gorse showed that the state of hopelessness followed a physical or emotional set-back or trauma. Both these remedies, Gorse and Hornbeam, relate to earthly existence, to the here and now. "The affairs of every day seem too much for them to accomplish, though they generally succeed in fulfilling their task." Hornbeam is the remedy to assist in overcoming both the Gentian and the Gorse states. Not everyone who experiences the Gentian discouragement will necessarily experience Gorse hopelessness.

Whilst most people do succeed in fulfilling their daily tasks, however little enthusiasm they may feel, there are occasions when the task is too great. I am not referring merely to an inability to complete a hoped for number of tasks in any one day, rather I am referring to an ongoing state, approaching that of a break-down. This situation does not come within the scope of Hornbeam and will be considered later when we study another remedy.

Hornbeam, then, is for the condition of lack of enthusiasm, when life becomes a drudge and there is no joy left in the anticipation of the daily round. It is said that Hornbeam has become known as 'the Monday morning feeling' remedy. It says much about our perception of the average person's attitude to their paid employment that such a term has come into the vernacular.

Remembering that this is the group of remedies for Uncertainty or Doubt, what is the uncertainty or doubt connected with Hornbeam? There are two main manifestations. The first is short-term. Do I have the strength and tenacity to carry on my daily task. The second is long-term. Am I following my appointed way? Is it time for a change?

Of course, nearly everyone will feel down in the dumps at the thought of 'another day at the office' at some time or another. This does not mean that they will seriously consider leaving for another employer or changing their career altogether, but if the state persists for some time, with total lack of enthusiasm, then these possibilities must be considered. Hornbeam may help clarify the issue, bringing either a return of interest in the task at hand or the energy to consider other options.

These options may be with regard to ill-health as well as daily living. It is the remedy to assist either the Gentian or the Gorse person to try again. While the former two remedies bring a change in outlook, Hornbeam helps the flow of energy into the physical body so that that which is necessary may be accomplished.

I spoke earlier of the boredom of the Scleranthus state, the boredom of inactivity through not knowing what to do. The boredom of Hornbeam occurs while knowing what to do, but finding the activity dull and uninspiring. I remember once hearing a preacher ask "Do you wake up in the morning and say, "Good morning, God" or "Good God, it's morning?" If your answer is the latter, add Hornbeam to the preacher's prescription of prayer!

Dr. Bach completed his indications for Hornbeam "For those that believe that some part of mind or body needs to be strengthened before they can easily fulfill their work". Consider Hornbeam arriving home from work, feeling tired and looking forward to a quiet evening in front of the television.

The telephone rings. A friend, not seen for years, is in town and wants to call round. Several hours later finds our Hornbeam friend full of energy, still talking nineteen-to-the-dozen. The body was quite capable of responding; all it needed was the mental/emotional stimulus. This belies Hornbeam's belief that they are too tired or too overworked. All they need to recapture their energy is enthusiasm from within (en — in; theos — God).

Hornbeam people cannot, and must not, wait each day for some external circumstances to enliven their life. Hornbeam will help to revive inner energies and to restore a sense of purpose.

True physical tiredness is a pleasant feeling, as anyone who sinks happily into a chair after a productive time spent working in the garden or playing an enjoyable sport, will know. To slip between the sheets at the end of a day during which the physical body has given well of its service, is to invite a peaceful and satisfying sleep. All unpleasant feelings of fatigue stem from the mind or the emotions, when we push ourselves too far or work at some undesired task. However, most people in a Hornbeam state will express their feeling of fatigue as physical. They feel tired and they are aware of this tiredness mostly in the way it affects the physical body.

Hornbeam is the first of four 'turning-point' remedies which we will discuss. This will become more clear later but, for now, suffice it to say that, during the Gorse stage, the soul could have chosen to withdraw, physically to have died by one means or another, which would have necessitated the cycle commencing all over again. This option was not chosen. The soul elected to stay on the physical plane to work out its destiny and Hornbeam is the remedy to bring strength to the soul to enable it to fulfill its daily round of duties in this material world.

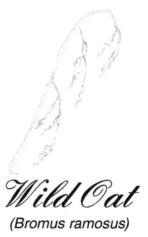

Wild Oat
(Bromus ramosus)

Of all the uncertainty or doubt remedies, Wild Oat is the most optimistic. Wild Oat is one of the grasses from which modern cereal crops have been derived. Many seeds hang from each stem and each one of them is potentially productive! This plant is used to harness potential energy and to direct it so that it may accomplish that which is of greatest benefit, both for the individual and the world.

Dr. Bach tells us that this is the remedy "for those who have ambitions to do something of prominence in life, who wish to have much experience, to enjoy all that is possible for them, to take life to the full. Their difficulty is to determine which occupation to follow. Although their ambitions are strong, they have no calling which appeals to them above all others."

Dr. Bach discovered this plant while seeking a remedy for those lacking direction in their lives, as lack of incentive could lead, not only to boredom with their daily duties, but also to a lack of desire to be well again when sick or injured.

We recognize the place Wild Oat takes following the boredom and lack of incentive of Hornbeam. Now the Hornbeam state is passing. Enthusiasm for life is returning. It is recognized that changes need to be made. The decision is taken to make them. But how? Where? When? In what direction? Unless the correct direction is found, not only will precious time and energy be lost, but the delay may cause dissatisfaction and the person may revert once again to the Cerato/ Scleranthus/Gentian state. Indeed, the whole cycle of the group may recur. The soul may not be able to step from the treadmill upon which it has imprisoned itself.

I spoke earlier of Scleranthus being a remedy often required in adolescence, when decisions needed to be made with regard to future directions in life. Wild Oat may also be required at this time. The child has grown, having reached the peak of its physical growth and fitness. The young are aware of their strength, they feel their potential. The world is their oyster. Now is the time for them to go forth and make their impression upon the world. This is a time of confidence. Self doubt is passed.

Alas, not all young people feel this sense of purpose or, if they do, they are unsure of the specific direction to take. Remember, Wild Oat is not indicated for those who have no idea at all of what they want to do; it is for those who have a number of interests and skills and who are finding it difficult to choose the best direction to follow.

People who achieve greatness usually do so in one area. This is not to say they are not skilled in many but, be they musicians, sportsmen, artists, scientists, they have one area of skill into which they direct most of their energies. Great achievements need concentration.

In each incarnation we need to direct the rays of our energies to accomplish a specific task. This task may not be one which receives public recognition. Tasks may also be non-material — to learn courage, patience, diligence, there are so many things to practice and achieve. When our energies are correctly focused, other qualities will take their rightful place and find their rightful expression.

Wild Oat is frequently needed at that stage referred to as 'mid-life crisis', which often occurs after many years of employment in a position which has become humdrum, which no longer offers much opportunity for expansion and learning, for which one has lost enthusiasm (Hornbeam) and where one has gathered enough life experience to feel able to branch out in a new, more challenging, direction. Mid-life is a time for reviewing, "What have I accomplished? Can I do something more fulfilling? And if so, what?"

Dr. Bach spoke of Wild Oat in another connection. It was one of two remedies he recommended for use when a number of flower remedies seemed indicated in the same person. This may be because the person's mental focus is not clear enough to perceive the underlying cause of their problem and to choose the remedy required. It may be that the practitioner is unable to focus clearly on the underlying cause. In such a case, it may be beneficial for both the patient and the practitioner to take Wild Oat.

Wild Oat may be of benefit to students, business people, busy mothers, anyone who has much on their mind, much which needs to be accomplished and who need to be able to focus their attention on the task in hand.

Retirement sees many a Wild Oat situation, especially in times of early retirement coupled with increased longevity.

Be aware of displaced dissatisfaction. It may well be that there is no awareness that a change of path is needed to bring a sense of true fulfillment. Instead, the sufferer may merely be aware of a state of inner restlessness which they may try to resolve by moving house, taking a holiday, changing the physical scenery in some way, when what is truly needed is a change of attitude from within.

As the first group concluded with its most outward looking remedy, so does the second. Wild Oat is bringing to a close a destructive pattern of self-doubt, replacing it with constructive confidence and certainty. The soul is now able to look outwards, to see and accept its role in the great cosmic drama.

This is an exciting time. The soul is on the threshold of great achievements. Now is the time to enjoy all that is possible, to take life to the full.

Of the seven positive soul qualities listed by Dr. Bach, Certainty is the antithesis of Uncertainty. That this quality was placed by Dr. Bach in his list of 'top seven' is itself food for thought.

Chapter Seven

Not Sufficient Interest in Present Circumstances
(Group Three)

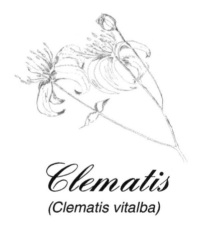

Clematis
(Clematis vitalba)

Traveller's Joy! What a beautiful remedy to start the next stage of our journey! And how well it follows the last remedy of the previous group, which was the remedy to help us enjoy all that is possible in life.

We left our soul on the verge of great things. But no great thing is ever accomplished without much thought and planning. Day-dreaming, planning, living in the world of ideas, these things are necessary for anyone with ambition, but they must not be overdone.

The Clematis plant itself is a climbing vine which needs another plant or structure to support it and it provides us with the remedy for those people who spend so much time reaching for the sky that they fail to keep their feet on the ground! A stereotypical Clematis personality would be that of the 'mad professor', shut in his laboratory with little or no interest in the world outside, engrossed in his own world of impractical ideas. As to the practicality of daily living, almost certainly that is the responsibility of his long-suffering wife!

To bring an idea to fruition, the first essential is to be practical.

Dr. Bach described the Clematis person as being dreamy, drowsy, not fully awake and, one could add, not fully alive. The new-born infant spends much of its time sleeping; as it grows older, it becomes more interested in its surroundings, exploring and experiencing. But the child's interest in its physical surroundings is off-set by its interest in the world of imagination. At times it may have difficulty establishing the boundary between imagination and reality, a task not made easier by the 'whoppers' told them by adults! All young children tell lies at times and deny being responsible for misdemeanours. Chronic liars may need Clematis to bring them back to reality.

Gradually, there needs to be an adjustment. For the Clematis person, this is not easy. They may continue to day-dream their way through school, not attending to their lessons, forgetting their homework, thinking only of the end of class time or school for the day. "Not really happy in the present circumstances, living more in the future than in the present. Living in hope of happier times, when their ideas may come true."

For these people, the grass is always greener on the other side of the street. There is little point in planning tomorrow's dinner if, in so doing, you are failing to enjoy the meal you have prepared for this day.

Clematis is one of the ingredients of Rescue Remedy, a combination of five remedies which Dr. Bach prepared for use in emergencies. The other four are Cherry Plum, Impatiens, Star of Bethlehem and Rock Rose. Clematis is the remedy for states of fainting, unconsciousness or concussion. This last condition combines two indications: loss of consciousness and loss of memory. Clematis is the first remedy to be considered for poor memory in people of all ages, especially if there is no apparent reason other than inattention to matters of daily life.

While we often think of young people dreaming of the future, we must not forget that elderly people may spend much time dreaming also. Dr. Bach specifically indicated that Clematis was for forward dreaming (not nostalgia), but he pointed out that sick or elderly people may look forward to death in the hope of better times ahead, especially if they are hoping to be reunited with some beloved one whom they have lost.

While sleep is essential for healing, and sick people do need to sleep a great deal, sleep can also be used as a means of escape from reality. If the person seems to be unnaturally unconcerned about their condition, as if a state of loss of interest is uppermost, it would not be out of order to administer some Clematis. No remedy of this type can retain a soul earthbound against its will. If the time has come for it to move on, Clematis will be of no avail, but if there is yet more for the soul to experience on this plane, then Clematis will refocus the attention.

Clematis is an important remedy for shock or grief. The first reaction of shock is one of disbelief: "This can't be happening". The person feels dazed, as if in a dream. This state does not last long, although it may return in a fluctuating manner, and Clematis is the appropriate remedy. Some people never recover from their shock or grief, whatever it may be, the loss of a loved one, a marriage, a home, a business, a dream.

Often Star of Bethlehem is routinely prescribed if there is a history of shock, grief, or other trauma. Clematis must not be overlooked, especially in cases where there is a loss of interest in life, a blank or vacant expression and/or resignation.

Some people report having 'out of body' experiences following accidents, shocks or operations. We are told that re-entry of the soul into the body remains possible so long as the silver cord, which emanates from the solar plexus, is in tact. Clematis is the main remedy which reinforces this link between the material and non-material aspects of our being.

Honeysuckle
(Lonicera caprifolium)

Honeysuckle is another climbing plant, but its use is opposite from that of Clematis, because it is for those who look back, for those who live much in the past. In the same way that Dr. Bach spoke of Clematis people living in hopes of happier times to come, he spoke of the Honeysuckle person thinking back to great happiness in times gone by.

One would think first of this remedy for people in later stages of life, looking back upon their childhood, upon their younger years, the prime of their life, as they slip into old age and, no doubt, Honeysuckle is frequently indicated in our Senior Citizens. However, Honeysuckle may be indicated at any stage once the ability to hold memories is sufficiently developed. A young child in its first year at school may well think back with longing to its time in kindergarten!

Children of separated or divorced parents often long to turn back the clock, for their parents to be reunited, for things to return to their former state. They may not express their feelings openly, not knowing in whom to confide. Changes in behavior (aggression, withdrawal) may indicate the need for this remedy.

Some may have experienced a happy childhood in a loving home, only to find adult life not so kind. An unhappy marriage, a difficult career path, financial difficulties not previously undergone, all these may lead to a feeling of nostalgia, a longing for past conditions and securities.

The remedy for homesickness or nostalgia (nostos — return home; algos — pain). For that feeling of not belonging, whether it be time or place.

Dr. Bach also spoke of "memories of a lost friend or ambitions, which have not come true". This shows another aspect of Honeysuckle: the memories may not always be pleasant. Memories of a lost friend may be happy or sad, depending on circumstances, but those of ambitions which have not come true must surely be tinged with sadness? The person may "recreate" in their mind scenarios once hoped for, never realized, but there will be a wistfulness to these past daydreams. During the Clematis time we were looking forward, planning. Now, some of our plans have gone awry and we are looking back with longing.

How we long to be able to turn back the clock, to live again those times, to make different decisions, to change outcomes. It is clear that this is a further remedy which may be of use at some stage in the process of grief.

Whether the memory is of a past event, or a dream which never eventuated, it is of a happiness gone by. Even in recalling a trauma, we are recalling the state of being before the trauma and we long to be able to recapture that state again. The hold of the past is preventing progress into the future.

The 'good old days' — how good they were — or were they? Many people in Western societies are exhibiting Honeysuckle tendencies in their cry "Back to Nature!" How many would truly wish to be without electricity, running water, plumbing, to say nothing of the telephone, electronic media and medical assistance? For a short time, yes. But permanently? How easy it is to deceive ourselves into thinking that life was easier or more pleasant in times gone by.

Memories are our most treasured possession. Time and again we pause along the way to dip into the well to drink once again of their nectar. Honeysuckle will help us grow by assimilating the experiences of the past without becoming entrapped by them. It will assist us to become more adaptable, to be open to change.

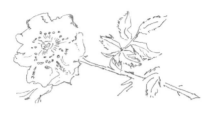

Wild Rose

(Rosa canina)

As we take up our study of Wild Rose, we find that a reaction has set in. The enthusiastic planning of the earlier remedies has dissipated in the face of the difficulties of life. The Honeysuckle state was one of backward looking, reliving past successes and regretting dreams and ambitions which had not eventuated. Now the soul feels like giving up. Things have not proceeded according to plan (they rarely do!) and Wild Rose has given up the fight.

Comparing Group 3, Wild Rose, with Group 2, Gentian, we see that the Gentian state of disheartenment was one which resulted from a known cause, whereas Wild Rose is indicated for those who, without sufficient reason, become resigned to all that happens.

Like the Mimulus state, Gentian related to known or worldly things (as do all the Group 2 remedies). Wild Rose is closer to Aspen, as are all the Group 3 remedies, because they relate to less tangible states.

Wild Rose touches a deeper level, because the despair is not merely in response to some obvious adversity of life, but stems from some sense of desperation which rises up from deep within the soul.

The depression from which the Wild Rose person suffers is somewhat different from the Gentian/Gorse person. They are less likely to grumble or complain, their attitude of compliance with whatever life dictates protecting them from that. However, the emptiness within is greater. They are also unlikely to be suicidal. It is as though they have not enough energy even for that. "They just glide through life, taking it as it is, without any effort to improve things and find some joy. They have surrendered to the struggle of life without complaint."

What brings a person to this state of apathy? It has been said that apathy represents suppressed or unacknowledged anger. Rather than hit out physically or verbally, they restrain themselves, consciously or subconsciously, and the destructive energy turns inwards, destroying the self. It may be that this is the better alternative, who is to say? Each life, and its circumstances, is different.

At times, the Wild Rose person may almost give the impression that they are pleased with themselves for having given up. "What will be, will be. It is fate, karma. Who am I to fight that which the wisdom of the Universe has decreed?"

"God give us the strength to change the things that need to be changed, the serenity to accept the things which cannot be changed, and the wisdom to know the difference." This prayer epitomizes the dilemma of Wild Rose — when does stoic endurance turn into resignation and weakness?

It seemed to me that some of my teenage children were exhibiting a strong Wild Rose state of apathy. While I worked long hours to keep a roof over our heads, they rarely cleaned their rooms, and even washing up a plate seemed to be a major hassle. One Friday night I slipped some Wild Rose into the milk. I arrived home Saturday lunch time to find that the Wild Rose had had an instant effect. My fourteen year-old daughter had decided to redecorate the house!

Having none of the required implements was not going to dampen her new found enthusiasm. Armed with her hair-dryer, she was melting the paint from the kitchen doors, using an old metal rule as a scraper! I learnt a lesson about medicating without consultation or consent! So, if you had your teenage children in mind, or even your husband, I urge you to think twice before slipping them a Wild Rose cocktail!

I leave you to ponder the ethical issue raised here. There is no easy answer. Whether or not love gives one the right to medicate another human being without their knowledge or consent, is a question which you must answer for yourself. How would you feel if someone else medicated you, without your knowledge?

Apathy can be yet another stage of grief. The derivation of the word 'apathy' is interesting: a - non; pathy — suffering. It is as though the mind adopts a state of neutrality in order to avoid feeling and, therefore, suffering. Dr. Bach did not use the word "apathy". He said "resigned", which means to relinquish or surrender, to hand over or give up.

Wild Rose offers us a hard lesson to learn, but a necessary one. There is not a soul which, at some stage or another of its existence, does not feel that the road is too long, the battle too hard, and who does not yearn to be able to surrender the struggle. But this is an option not vouchsafed to us. Life has to go on, whether on this plane or another. Wild Rose brings strength and courage to carry on with a greater sense of purpose and enthusiasm.

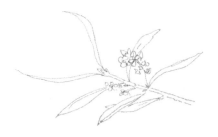

Olive
(Olea europæa)

In the second group of remedies we found the two states of discouragement and hopelessness were followed by a turning-point remedy, Hornbeam. And so it is with the third group. Following the resignation of Wild Rose, we find our second pick-me-up remedy, Olive, but this remedy has a far deeper action than that of Hornbeam, as is appropriate to its place following the far deeper state to which Wild Rose corresponded.

Although a number of the flowers selected by Dr. Bach were not indigenous to the British Isles, most were either native or had established themselves there in the wild. Only two remedies were obtained by Dr. Bach from overseas, Olive and Vine, both plants from Mediterranean countries, both plants which had grown in the Holy Land, although Dr. Bach's samples were not obtained from there.

Who can consider Olive and not be reminded of the Mount of Olives upon which Christ prayed the night before he passed over, the day before the Passover? Olive is the remedy for "those who have suffered much mentally or physically and are so exhausted and weary that they feel they have no more strength to make any more effort." Did the account of the 'Agony in the Garden' guide Dr. Bach to this remedy? We will never know.

When considering Hornbeam, it was pointed out that the Hornbeam exhaustion was more of the mind than of the body. If a suitable mental stimulus was forthcoming, the Hornbeam person would respond. The Olive person, not so. The person needing Hornbeam tends to brighten up as the day goes by; they draw energy from, and are stimulated by, people and events around them. The person needing Olive tends to become more tired as the day progresses.

Rather than drawing energy from people, they are drained and become more exhausted. Whereas the person needing Hornbeam usually equates their tiredness with the physical body, the person in need of Olive is fully aware that their exhaustion comes from deep within. This state is truly the result of mental stress. Olive helps to restore, not only physical energy, but mental interest in life — hence its placement after Wild Rose.

The apathy of Wild Rose may reach a state of non-feeling. There is no reserve of energy to respond to stimulii, be they of pleasure or pain. In a similar manner, the Olive person lacks reactive ability. Dr. Bach completed his description by saying "Daily life is hard work for them, without pleasure", showing that these people have now reached the stage of complete breakdown. They are able to undertake their daily work, but it is completed from necessity or duty. They may describe themselves as being exhausted to the point of tears.

I spoke of the person in the Wild Rose state being unlikely to commit suicide. They may too apathetic or tired to think or plan such a step, except possibly the swallowing of too many sleeping pills. The Olive state is one in which suicide is an option. As energy returns, the possibility of such a plan being made and executed increases. If the soul elects this path, then it must make its journey again. If not, then it will need the strength to carry on.

The Olive person may be described as being in a state of adrenal exhaustion. On the physical plane, undoubtedly they are. The answer to their underlying problem is not a shot of adrenalin, but a course of Olive to allow the soul's energy system to be recharged from a higher level.

Looking back, we see that the role of Wild Oat was to help people "take life to the full". Dr. Bach said that Olive was found to be the remedy for "those people who lived their lives to the full". We understand that the soul in the Olive state has not necessarily deviated from its path, but may have become too intense, possibly not taking enough time for rest and recreation (re-creation).

Considering this remedy within the context of the typical life span, it must surely correspond more to middle age, because the Olive state takes time to develop. One does not reach a state of adrenal exhaustion overnight. Middle age is that time when one has been endeavouring for a goodly number of years, not only on behalf of oneself, but frequently on behalf of one's family also. At this age society does not permit one to retire. There are many more years of struggle ahead before that option becomes viable. Physically, the body has passed its peak. Mentally, there may be further accomplishments yet possible.

Olive will help us succeed, whatever our task may be.

In considering these remedies, we need to remember that not all souls go through all states every incarnation, or within the period of one life episode. For example, just because one has a new idea (Clematis) does not mean that one will necessarily be found some time later in a Wild Rose state of apathy or an Olive state of exhaustion. Also, one may reach the Olive state of exhaustion without previously experiencing the Wild Rose state of apathy. Nevertheless, I do believe that we must all experience every state many, many times during the course of our individual evolution as each soul manifests its part in the greater evolution of the Soul of mankind.

While we may not know what prompted Dr. Bach to send abroad for this remedy, we do know that the Olive tree flowers, fruits and flourishes beneath the warmth of the Mediterranean sun.

Dr. Bach proved that the flower of the Olive tree contained the life, warmth and strength to re-energise such people. It would appear that for this state, much greater warmth or heat was required than could be obtained beneath the cooler British sun. This is the remedy to restore lost energy to the solar (sun) plexus and its associated organs (Weeks 1942).

Olive has ever been the symbol of peace. After the Flood, a dove brought a sprig of olive to Noah as a sign that the worst was over. It was the signal to step forth once more into the world. It was the symbol of regeneration.

Olive brings with it the dual blessing of strength for the tired body and peace for the tired mind.

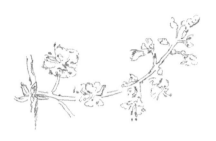

White Chestnut

(Æsculus hippocastanum)

This is the second of the four remedies which Dr. Bach drew from the family of Chestnut, which shows how powerful these trees must be. Two are found in this, the third group, White Chestnut and Chestnut Bud. The latter is the bud of the former. Children know this tree for its gift of the horse chestnut, with which they delight to play the time-honoured game of 'conkers'.

Inability to fix attention is the greatest characteristic of the White Chestnut flower, for this is the remedy for those who cannot control their thoughts.

Olive brought a return of energy to the person exhausted in body and mind. Energy is returning, but it would be naïve to assume that all such people immediately return to a state of productivity. Many will still feel at a loss, dissatisfied with their present situation but not yet feeling themselves to be in a position to make a positive change. During this time, the eddies and swirls of returning energy lack direction.

We remember that this third group of remedies is for those with not sufficient interest in present circumstances. Dr. Bach told us that the principle use of White Chestnut was for those occasions when the interest of the moment was not strong enough to keep the mind full. This is an important statement, as it helps us to distinguish between White Chestnut, Agrimony and Crab Apple. The tormenting nature of the White Chestnut unwanted thoughts lies in their triviality — they are unproductive. White Chestnut helps us direct our attention to the task in hand, whatever this may be.

It is hard at times to concentrate on small tasks, to give them our full attention, but of such is life composed. The greatest athletes, the greatest musicians, the greatest artists, the greatest achievers in any sphere of life, are not performing all the time. Their days are spent practising and practising the small details of their craft upon which are built their great achievements. It is the ability to focus, even during times of repetitive, routine activity, which separates the champion from the rest. In the White Chestnut state, there is an inability of the mind to control its thoughts, thoughts which are not those of major life events or of big decisions, but those of useless trivia, which go round and round in the brain, tormenting the sufferer who is completely unable to assert any authority over them. If one cannot control one's thoughts, how can one expect to control anything else?

It is not only worrying thoughts which are difficult to control. Over-activity of the mind also occurs in anticipation of, or following, some enjoyable events and White Chestnut may be needed if such thoughts monopolize the attention to the exclusion of the more mundane tasks of life which, nevertheless, must be completed. The 'task' may be to sleep. All the hard practice may be to no avail if the player turns up for the match tired out from lack of sleep!

"For those who cannot prevent thoughts, ideas, arguments which they do not desire from entering their minds." These thoughts, ideas, arguments, may be anticipatory in nature or they may be the reworking of some past event. Such reworkings are not entirely useless. We learn a great deal by mentally reviewing our thoughts and actions, judging those times when we have performed well and rehearsing our less satisfactory performances with a view to doing better next time. This mental rehearsing should not dominate our life. With some people, it does.

Such uncontrolled thoughts drive out peace; that peace of mind we fought so hard to achieve in our Olive state. In fact, it is possible to experience the Olive and the White Chestnut states together. Continued thoughts may lead to insomnia, which will aggravate the mental and physical exhaustion of Olive. Similarly, overwork, which precipitates the Olive exhaustion, may lead to the White Chestnut state of mind, where one lies awake at night, thinking and thinking over the problems of yesterday and tomorrow, instead of sinking into a deep and peaceful sleep, which should be the pleasure of 'now'.

The Clematis state was characterized by an enjoyment of the world of thought. The White Chestnut person dreads their thoughts, not necessarily because of their unpleasant nature, but because they cannot escape from them. To the Clematis or Honeysuckle person, thoughts are a haven; to the White Chestnut person they are a hell.

Thoughts are seeds. They who are in control of their thoughts may plan that which their heart desires. They who cannot control their thoughts must accept the seeds which the passing breeze blows into their garden, or that which is dropped therein by the winged elements, which flutter through on their way to other pastures. There were no weeds in the Garden of Eden, because a weed is a plant out of place. When the mind is cleared of unwanted thoughts, there will be no weeds in the Garden of the Mind, and no weeds in the Garden of the Soul.

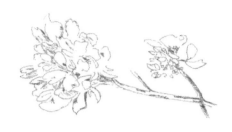

Mustard
(Sinapis arvensis)

With White Chestnut, Dr. Bach spoke of unpleasant thoughts, which drove out peace and prevented the sufferers from being able to think of the work and pleasures of that day. From there, he proceeded to Mustard, where unpleasant or dark thoughts no longer merely swirled around in the mind, they took control and completely dominated it. Both the White Chestnut and the Mustard person are, to a large extend, prisoners of their mind. They cannot release themselves from the bondage of their thoughts.

Dr. Bach spoke of these people as being overshadowed by a cold, dark cloud which hid the light and joy of life. These are words typically used by persons suffering endogenous depression in an attempt to portray their suffering. Dr. Bach was writing for lay people. He did not use the words 'endogenous depression' but there can be no doubt about that of which he was speaking because he goes on to say that it may not be possible for these people to give any reason or explanation for such attacks.

'Endogenous' means 'coming from within' in contrast to

exogenous' meaning 'coming from without,' which term is used to describe depression developing in response to adverse life events, also known as 'reactive' depression. We have already studied the remedy for this latter state (Gorse).

Those suffering from reactive depression are able to offer some explanation for their state and, therefore, to retain some feeling of control in their life. Even if the precipitating cause of their depression was an event outside their control, such as the death of a loved one, they can see a progression of cause and effect which helps them make some sense of their situation. Even though they may be reluctant to admit it, somewhere deep within their hearts they know that life does go on, that time will bring a measure of healing, that one day they will smile again, even if somewhat tearfully.

The person suffering from endogenous depression does not have even that small glimmer of comfort. They cannot account for their state and, therefore, they cannot look forward to any promise of its cessation.

Like the White Chestnut person before them, the Mustard people have no control over their thoughts, or state of mind, however unwelcome. At times they may feel quite normal, or even over cheerful. If extreme, this latter state is called 'manic', and persons suffering from 'manic-depression' (bi-polar disorder) swinging from states of uncontrolled enthusiasm, rapid thought, speech and action to states of depression, would clearly benefit from White Chestnut and Mustard alternately, depending on the state manifesting at any particular time.

I would point out that manic-depression is a serious psychological disturbance and that such a person should be under the care of a qualified psychotherapist or other medical practitioner. Fortunately, the Bach Flower remedies do not interfere with orthodox medication and the sufferer may take both treatments concurrently, if so desired.

Many people suffer from depression with no apparent manic episodes although at times the black cloud will lift and life will seem good again. For these people, Mustard alone may be the only Bach Flower remedy indicated.

A further guide to the difference between exogenous (Gorse) and endogenous (Mustard) depression is that the Gorse person can make an effort to be cheerful for a while if the social situation demands it. It may be only their family and close friends who understand something of the depth of their suffering. The Mustard person finds it far more difficult to dissemble. As Dr. Bach so rightly said: "Under these conditions it is almost impossible to appear happy or cheerful".

It is important to point out that it is of no avail to say to these people "Pull yourself together. There are other people worse off than you." They know this and the knowledge only adds to their suffering. They cannot help themselves. If they could, they would not be suffering endogenous depression. They may say, "I have a loving spouse, beautiful family, am financially secure, yet I feel utterly depressed. Please help me." Maybe Mustard can.

Our subconscious is a powerful, bottomless reservoir of emotions and desires, many of which are suppressed from our normal waking consciousness, although they may make their presence known in our dreams. At times, the build up of these suppressed thoughts and emotions becomes so great that their cold, dark shadow emerges from the depths of our subconscious mind and manifests into our waking consciousness as endogenous depression. While only a small proportion of the population is destined to suffer the torments of this form of depression in any one life time, yet surely each one of us will, at some stage of our evolution, need to come to grips with the dark suppressed side of our nature, to acknowledge and learn the lessons we have tried so hard to bury, hide, ignore and deny.

Let us not forget that growth takes place in darkness. The seed must needs be buried in the earth before it can grow. The baby develops and grows within the darkness of the womb. Each night Nature clothes us with a blanket of darkness and we sink into the blessed oblivion of sleep, while our bodies repair themselves after the ravages of the day and our dream time allows our mind the opportunity to review, process and absorb the lessons of the day's events and to make itself ready for the dawning of the morrow.

The darkness may be deepest before the dawn, but dawn always comes.

Chestnut Bud
(Æsculus hippocastanum)

And so does Spring, bringing with it the promise of better things to come.

Within the confines of the sticky bud of the White Chestnut tree it was that Dr. Bach discovered the remedy to release the tortured mind from the prison created by its thoughts.

Chestnut Bud is the remedy to help us take full advantage of life's experiences, to learn life's lessons, to save us from unnecessary repetition of errors. Mustard helped us come face to face with our shadow side, to convert its negative energies into growth potential. Now Chestnut Bud will help us open into full bloom.

This is the last remedy of the third group and, once again, we finish with a note of optimism. The person who is experiencing the Chestnut Bud state may not feel very optimistic, because repeated mistakes and failings will bring repeated problems, but the point to be held in mind in studying this remedy is that the soul has now reached the stage where it is capable of learning life's lessons and of reaping the benefit.

This remedy will enable one to leave behind negative thoughts and patterns which are holding one back. In his gentle manner, Dr. Bach said: "Whereas one experience would be enough for some, such people find it necessary to have more, sometimes several, before the lesson is learnt." Maybe there are some people who learn life's lessons after only one try, but I doubt there would be many. It has been said that within the classroom we retain only about five per cent of the knowledge imparted. The teacher needs to repeat the points being made and the student to restudy and revise their notes for an acceptable level of assimilation to take place. If this is true of the classroom, how much more must it be true in the school of life? Indeed, why else would we need to incarnate again and again if it were not to learn our lessons more completely?

This remedy may be of service within the schoolroom for the child who, quite literally, needs to repeat a lesson several times before it is learned. Later in life, it may help those who repeatedly form friendships with unsuitable people, even marry unsuitable partners, on successive occasions. Inability to shed childish habits, temper outbursts, immature language as well as comfort eating and drinking, all may need the help of Chestnut Bud.

Repeated lessons. Repeated accidents. Repeated situations. Repeated illnesses. Some ailments are cyclical by nature, such as hay fever — or manic depression - others keep recurring, such as headaches. While some people can drive for years accident free, others have repeated bingles, not necessarily serious but enough to cause one to wonder why? Repeated financial difficulties or job losses. Some lesson is needing to be presented again and again.

We note that Dr. Bach started his description of Chestnut Bud by speaking of taking full advantage of observations and experience. He concluded by speaking of observations of others which could have spared even that one fault. Not until the end does he slip in the word 'fault' — fault being groove, imperfection, defect or blemish. And truly, repeated lessons are our 'fault'.

Observation and experience. Observation of others — and of the self! Merely observing others is of no use unless the observations be turned into experience within the self.

In some ways, this is a regrouping remedy, a remedy for those who are assimilating life's experiences, are preparing to move ahead to another level. This will become more clear as we study the remedies in the next group.

Chestnut Bud acts within this group in a similar manner to that of Wild Oat in the last. It pulls everything together. It is as if it were saying: "Very well. What have you been through? What was the purpose of your experience? Do you want to go through the same experience again? Or have you learnt your lesson? If not, very well, we will recycle it again for you." It is a time for re-assessing where you are, where you have come from, where you are going, what you have learnt, what you have yet to learn, why you need to keep repeating certain things, why do certain things keep happening to you?

The third group of remedies has born some resemblance to the second. Both started with remedies of an uncertain or dreamy nature, both descended into despondency or depression, both received help in the form of a physical or emotional tonic, both ended with a remedy of promise. The difference between the two groups is that the former corresponded more to physical or earthly experiences, while the latter groups corresponded to less tangible states.

Chestnut Bud brings this group full circle. From the dreams of youthful Clematis, we have now reached the realization of lessons learned and yet to be learned. The idealism of youth is giving way to the wisdom of maturity.

Of the seven positive soul qualities mentioned by Dr. Bach, I believe Joy to be the one which relates to this group. The scene was set with the first remedy, Traveller's Joy, and it is ever present joy that is so desperately needed by the souls experiencing the state of growth corresponding to this group's flowers.

Chapter Eight

Loneliness
(Group Four)

Water Violet
(Hottonia palustris)

Water Violet is the first of only three remedies which form this, the shortest, of all the groups.

Dr. Bach tells us that this is the remedy for the person who likes to be alone, for the person who moves through life quietly and gently. They are often clever and talented and their peace and calmness is a blessing to those around them. They are independent, capable and self-reliant, almost free of the opinion of others.

So pleasing is Dr. Bach's description of these people that the question is invariably asked: "Why do they need a remedy?" There are two reasons. Even people of this personality type do become ill and need treatment. Secondly, they do have some faults. For example, they tend to be aloof and, at times, proud.

The Eastern religions have taken the lotus, or Water Lily, as the symbol of enlightenment. It rises from the earthly mud (of materialism) through the water (of emotions) ever striving to break through, to reach the clear light of day. At last it blossoms in the full sun of spirituality, where it sits at peace with itself and its surroundings. The humble Water Violet, too, strives to rise above the waters (of emotions), standing tall and proud in its self-sufficiency. However, the Water Violet state is not that of the perfection symbolized by the lotus. The Water Violet person has learnt to be independent, to go their own way, and this is good, but at times they may be aloof and unapproachable, they may feel superior to those around them. They may fail to aid and assist their fellow beings, taking the attitude, "If I can stand alone, why cannot they?"

The Water Violet child often seems to possess a wisdom beyond its years. Like Water Violet people of all ages, they seem to be secure in the knowledge that they have a right to be here.

Meditation comes naturally to the self-contained Water Violet people. They are contemplative, happy to live alone and, therefore, likely to marry late. They are listeners, rather than talkers, and may attract to themselves people who need solace and understanding. However, their quiet, attentive attitude may be deceiving. While prepared to listen for politeness' sake, they may be short in offers of practical help. Because of their inherent self-sufficiency, Water Violet people do not often seek help for themselves, preferring to fight their own battles.

Even in sickness, they will be reluctant to consult a

therapist, or even to mention their complaint at home. They will bear pain with less complaint than any other remedy, with the possible exception of Rock Water. (The two 'water' remedies both tend to be independent and stoical.)

The Water Violet types are not necessarily reclusive. They are quite happy to be in company provided that company does not make demands upon them. They do not interfere with others and they do not expect others to interfere with them.

Water Violet people tend to prefer individual sports, such as tennis, golf, single sailing, to team sports. Likewise, their hobbies tend to be unusual and individualistic. They may devote hours to stamp collecting, or the collection, arranging and cataloguing of unusual items. They may be interested in archæology, having the patience for the hours of careful digging and scraping which may be necessary to uncover even a single item.

Whereas Chestnut Bud failed to take full advantage of observation and experience, and thus was slow to learn the lessons of life, Water Violet is an astute observer. Whereas Chestnut Bud tended to act without thinking, Water Violet tends to think without acting. They believe that quality is superior to quantity in both thought and action.

Chestnut Bud and Water Violet both tend to 'wall off' from other people's experience and may fail to make completely satisfactory personal relationships.

Water Violet takes its place as the first of the remedies for Loneliness because these people travel their road alone by choice. At times they may appear to wish to alienate themselves from the rest of humanity. The Water Violet soul is learning to enjoy its independence but at the same time it must remember not to close its heart towards its fellow travelers on the Path.

Intermission

Water Violet was the nineteenth of the thirty-eight remedies which we have to study. We have reached the half-way point of our journey. Much has been undertaken. Much has been accomplished. Much has been learnt. How far we have come from the terror of Rock Rose with which our journey commenced! Now the soul feels secure. It has matured and feels capable of traveling alone.

You will recall that at the end of Chapter Four, I spoke of Dr. Bach's belief that the first nineteen of the remedies he discovered related in some way to the second nineteen, that he started working out this relationship but never completed this task. I went on to say that I believed that there was indeed a primary and a secondary group, each of nineteen remedies. I believe that we have just completed the first group and that the second nineteen we are about to study express a different aspect of the energy represented by the remedy from the first group with which it is paired.

It was not the first nineteen remedies which Dr. Bach found which were paired with the last nineteen. It was the first nineteen remedies which Dr. Bach presented which were to be paired with the last nineteen.

The soul goes forth. The soul returns to its source again. We have followed its outward journey; now it is time to follow its journey home.

As the first group of nineteen remedies opened with a remedy which was full of nervous energy, so does the second.

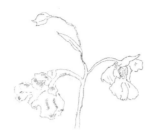

Impatiens
(Impatiens glandulifera)

Impatiens was the first remedy discovered by Dr. Bach and, not surprisingly, it is one to which he felt related. Although found growing wild among the Welsh mountains, it is native to Kashmir.

This is the remedy for "Those who are quick in thought and action and who wish all things to be done without hesitation or delay." Dr. Bach does not here mention speech, but these people also speak quickly and may even interrupt another's sentence once they have deduced its likely conclusion, so that they may respond without delay.

There is probably no greater example of concentration than the diver poised at the end of the diving board. He gathers together his total energies, physical, mental and emotional, and achieves a state of perfect stillness. And then! He launches himself forth into an intricate pattern of twists and turns, manœvering his body so fast that only the trained eye can follow the brilliance of his performance. There can be no better illustration of the relationship between Water Violet and Impatiens than this.

Whilst those trained in the art of diving are able to appreciate the diver in action, many others find it necessary to await the slow-motion replay fully to appreciate the standard of performance. And to the Impatiens person, this is the way the rest of the world appears — as a slow-motion replay. They, themselves, are so full of energy and enthusiasm, so eager to progress, that they find it hard to be patient with people who are slower than they. "They consider it wrong and a waste of time", said Dr. Bach, "and they will endeavor to make such people quicker in all ways".

There is nothing wrong with being quick in thought and action. The problem comes when such quickness brings in its wake feelings of impatience, intolerance, or even arrogance.

Dr. Bach concludes his short passage by saying that these people often prefer to work and think alone, so that they can do everything at their own speed.

Self-sufficiency has its advantages and its disadvantages — as we discovered when studying Water Violet. Being too efficient can lead to a tendency to reject help and assistance from others. Those whose offers of help have been rejected may feel that they have been rejected personally. Their self-esteem may be wounded, particularly if the rejection has come from some person in authority, such as a parent or employer, if it relates to some important project or if it is repeated many times in relation to smaller matters.

Nor is it only rejection of help which presents a lesson for the Impatiens soul. They also have a strong tendency to take over tasks that other people are undertaking, even if that task has no direct relationship to the work in which they are currently engaged. Merely seeing someone else working more slowly than they, can bring with it an irresistible desire to interfere, whether the recipient of this gratuitous assistance appreciates it or not. Incidentally, the word 'interference' comes from the Latin 'ferio' — to strike, and interference from another, more impatient, human being, while we are endeavouring to perform some task to the best of our ability, can be felt as a blow to our confidence and our self-esteem.

We see, then, how important it is that the Impatiens soul learns to be receptive to offers of help, from whatever source they may come. "I can do it quicker myself" — every parent alive must have had that thought at some stage as their youngster struggled to achieve some skill, be it tying their shoe laces or peeling the potatoes for dinner. Our love for our children prevents us from interfering (at least, not too often) as we appreciate their endeavour and understand their need to struggle to grow.

If we were to love others as we love our own family, we would extend to them the same courtesy of patience. How, then, are we to distinguish our desire to help from a desire to interfere? Help stems from the heart and is guided by wisdom.

Impatiens people are often of high intelligence. They are frequently more efficient than their peers in many ways but their inherent potential is no greater than that of any other soul, whatever its current stage of development.

Like White Chestnut, Impatiens must be considered for states of mania. A person in a state of mania believes that they are more intelligent, more perceptive, in possession of greater ideas, than other people. This is a temporary state, usually followed by depression. I repeat my earlier warning that mania is a serious disorder which should be treated by a qualified psychotherapist.

"When ill, they are anxious for a hasty recovery", not because they fear death or disease, but because they see it as a waste of time. Remembering how Dr. Bach worked day and night to complete his work when he believed he had only a short time to live, helps us to understand why he considered this to be his own remedy.

While Dr. Bach discouraged the attachment of specific physical conditions to any remedy, nevertheless he used Impatiens at times for patients suffering pain, and this seems a reasonable prescription based merely on mental characteristics. Anyone experiencing pain is impatient for its cessation and so, too, one would presume, are the suffering tissues! (For intense, unbearable pain, remember also Cherry Plum.)

Although Impatiens people normally have plenty of energy to complete their daily work, the one thing which will tire them out is frustration. If they cannot get on, that is hard to bear.

It is said that the vibrational rate of the more spiritually evolved Beings is higher than ours — that it is difficult for them to lower their vibrations to make contact with us. Similarly, humans developing spiritually, moving on towards a higher level of understanding, begin to operate at a higher rate and find it difficult to tolerate the coarser vibrations of average humanity. Our developing soul, starting its journey homewards, is experiencing a raising of its vibrational rate. In the Water Violet state, it may choose to retire to the Himalayas (literally or metaphorically). In the Impatiens state, it will choose to work within the world, although it will find this difficult at times.

We see that, like Water Violet, Impatiens is included under remedies for Loneliness because these people prefer to be, or to work, alone.

If Dr. Bach believed that he exhibited Impatiens characteristics, we can surely claim with confidence that he also manifested positive Water Violet traits. Both Water

Violet and Impatiens are independent people. Water Violet is independent in thought, Impatiens is independent in action. During his solitary walks in the countryside, his hours of silent meditation, Dr. Bach was manifesting the Water Violet side of his nature, for these are the natural proclivity of those of the Water Violet type. After his meditations, he was impatient to complete his work and for the knowledge he had attained to be spread abroad amongst suffering humanity, and this is the province of Impatiens. For a successful outcome, thought must precede action.

You will have noticed that throughout this section I have repeatedly compared Water Violet with Impatiens. Although at first glance they may appear to be completely different from each other, closer consideration shows that their underlying fault is the same. It is a feeling of superiority, of being better than others, of aloofness or pride.

I believe these two remedies are manifesting different aspects of the same negative state. In the one state, the person tends to be introverted, in the other extroverted. The same person may fluctuate between the two manifestations, as surely did Dr. Bach. These two remedies form the first of the nineteen pairs.

Heather

(Calluna vulgaris)

Heather is one of the 'Four Helpers' and we are told that Dr. Bach was guided to its use by asking someone, whom he described as being self-centred and utterly worldly, what was her favourite flower?

In his booklet, Dr. Bach described Heather as being for "Those who are always seeking the companionship of anyone who may be available, as they find it necessary to discuss their own affairs with others, no matter whom they may be. They are very unhappy if they have to be alone for any length of time".

It immediately becomes apparent that the loneliness of Heather is completely different from that of either Water Violet or Impatiens. These people are truly lonely because they dread loneliness and yet so often this is their lot.

Like Impatiens before them, the Heather type talks rapidly, but incessantly, and their favourite topic of conversation is themselves. They tend to stand close to the person to whom they are speaking and bombard them with their news, no matter how trivial, and leave their listener sapped of energy.

In contrast to Water Violet, Heather is a poor listener. Of all the remedies, Water Violet is the most tolerant towards Heather people. They will allow the Heather chatter to pass them by, while they mentally withdraw. Centaury will find it difficult to assert themselves sufficiently to escape Heather's attentions but within themselves they will be fretting and fuming as they will be less able to 'switch off' from the verbal onslaught and escape to another world.

While there seem to be some people who are born Heathers, all of us experience Heather states at one time or another. Listen to the teenage girl talking about her latest boy-friend! Or, worse still, listen to her after her relationship has ended! Whether it be the excitement of something new, or the disappointment of something lost, there are times when we all need to be able to pour out our feelings to a sympathetic ear. Before or after an operation, before or after a Court appearance, there are so many life experiences that seem to dominate our thoughts to such an extent that we are unable to put them aside sufficiently to take a genuine interest in the affairs of others.

It is understandable that Heather should take its place after Impatiens because a new interest fills us with enthusiasm and impatience to start. While the new interest is the centre of our attention, there may be a tendency to adopt a Heather attitude towards our long suffering friends. This 'interest' may be a new business, or an expansion of an existing one. Heather may manifest as much in the world of business and finance as at home 'over the fence'.

Another remedy which we will be studying later, Vervain, has a similar state, the difference being that Heather is only interested in issues relating to their own welfare, while the Vervain person is enthusiastic about issues relating to the welfare of humanity at large.

An interesting case is presented by Weeks in The Medical Discoveries of Edward Bach, Physician. It is that of a man who was of a jovial type, most happy when surrounded by companions to whom he could talk, apt to speak much about his own affairs and health. This is the only place I know where something positive is said about the Heather person! At least he is described as being 'jovial'. Small though this indication is, yet I feel it to be important. In their own way, they are outgoing — they do enjoy the company of other human beings. It is a pity that their self-centredness deprives them so often of the company which they so much desire. If these people can be kept physically occupied in some good work (because they do like to help where they can), then their willingness to serve others will help transmute self-love into selfless love.

And Heather's partner? I believe this to be Chestnut Bud. Both these remedies demonstrate an inability to listen and to learn from others. Chestnut Bud relates to the need to learn the lessons of daily life, to learn to listen, to watch, to understand the workings of the world. Heather needs to learn to listen to people, to watch, to be aware of and to understand their wants and needs.

Of the seven positive soul qualities listed by Dr. Bach, I believe Love to be the antithesis of Loneliness. "Real love must be the utter forgetfulness of self."

Chapter Nine

Oversensitive to influences and ideas
(Group Five)

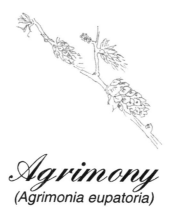

Agrimony
(*Agrimonia eupatoria*)

While few people will enjoy being described as Heather type, equally few will object to being described as Agrimony, for these people are cheerful and generally considered good friends to know. They hide their cares and worries behind a mask of cheerfulness, in total contrast to the Heather people, who cannot wait to unburden themselves upon anyone willing to listen.

Both Heather and Agrimony seek companionship, Heather to talk about their worries, Agrimony to escape from them.

Both have difficulty processing and assimilating life experiences. The one processes their experiences at night and alone, the other during the day and in company.

Society admires and tolerates so much better the Agrimony type yet, despite their many friends, they may suffer far more. Agrimony are learning to subjugate their own emotions in the interest of the greater good. For this reason, they have been placed later in the overall schema.

I spoke of the reaction of the Heather type to a broken relationship, of how they will verbalize at great length to whomsoever they can. Under similar circumstances, the Agrimony person will say little, but they may suffer as deeply, or even more so.

When the Agrimony people weep, they weep in private. Because Agrimony has become so expert at presenting a cheerful countenance to the world, they are often difficult to distinguish in practice. They do not speak out. Watch for these people; they often betray their inner state by their physical restlessness.

Dr. Bach described the Agrimony person as jovial, cheerful and humorous. The Agrimony person uses humour to deflect attention from their own concerns. They displace their own inner torment by telling jokes about other peoples' difficulties. By laughing at some other (hypothetical) person's discomfiture, Agrimony are helped in the working through of their own problems.

Night is a bad time for the Agrimony person. During the hours of darkness, they can no longer escape the burden of their thoughts. They endeavor not to worry other people with their troubles and during the day they are able to present a cheerful façade. As the shadows of darkness slip across the land, they bring no comforting blanket to an Agrimony tormented soul. As like welcomes like, so the shadows of the night call to the shadow side of Agrimony.

To help maintain their cheerful charade, a number of avenues are open to Agrimony. One is to keep busy, especially in the company of other people with whom they can converse, preferable about the other person's problems. (No wonder they are so popular!) When not at work, they can socialize through sporting and other activities — anything which delays the onset of the long, silent hours of the night. Another avenue open to them is the use of stimulants. Dr. Bach mentions alcohol or drugs, legal or illegal, in excess. In this group must be listed both coffee and cigarettes.

The Agrimony person is acting their way through life pretending that all is well with their world. The show must go on, even if their heart is breaking. In many ways, these are brave people, but at times they may compromise their integrity for the sake of peace. Dr. Bach tells us that they love peace and are distressed by argument or quarrel to avoid which they will agree to give up much. They will give way to another person's needs or desires rather than fight for their own. They may even give way on some point upon which they should not, or say the comfortable thing when they should have said the right thing.

Such loss of integrity may later haunt or torment them during their hours of reflection. There are times to be pacifist; there are times to stand up and fight.

Agrimony will make light of their concerns; when ill or before an operation they will joke with their attendants. Elderly people may hide their fear of death. Poor sleep patterns may result from a sub-conscious fear of allowing oneself to sink into unconsciousness lest one fail to awake.

I remember my very first Bach Flower prescription. I happened to be talking one day to someone whom I had known for some years. She was an outgoing, friendly person, well-liked among our circle of acquaintances. Her son was due to attend his first school camp the following week and she was anxious about his being away from home. She was joking about the up-coming event, of course, but it was only then that she confided that she had lost two daughters, both of whom died while young from an incurable hereditary disease.

Never before had I heard her mention these traumatic events, which threw such a different light upon her anxiety. Without this knowledge, I might have mistaken her fear for that of Red Chestnut. I gave her some Agrimony and next day received a telephone call telling me that she had felt the remedy act immediately, warming her from within. Not only was she able to wave 'Goodbye' to her son the following week without tears, she even looked forward to his departure so that she could take the opportunity to redecorate his room!

One of the privileges granted to those of us who work as therapists is that of being taken into the confidence of an Agrimony person. One comes to realize just how many there are of these courageous people. Rarely do they regard themselves as brave. They may be as easily deceived by the façade of their fellow Agrimony types as are the rest of us and this adds to their torment, for they feel they should be doing even better.

How easily are we misled by the superficial greetings of our friends and acquaintances! How easily we learn to exchange banalities!

Following the stock market crash of 1987 and the Global Financial Crisis of 2008, we saw more than the usual number of businesses go into liquidation, their owners facing financial ruin. Many people lost their employment.

Some sank into the state of disheartenment, despondency and apathy of which we have already spoken, others became jealous, bitter or revengeful, states which we will discuss shortly. Others still managed to smile. This illustrates Dr. Bach's principle of paying attention to the manner in which the patient has responded to any particular situation, rather than to the situation itself.

Agrimony takes its place alongside others, of which we have already spoken, for the state of grief. In this case, the people appear to be coping well, almost too well.

The Agrimony suicide is the suicide which takes others by surprise.

There is no doubt that Agrimony people are good friends to have. They are cheerful, rarely complain, and strive for peace. These positive attributes will be untouched by the administration of Agrimony. Any Bach Flower remedy will only transmute the negative, never negate the positive. It will help the Agrimony person to differentiate between the time to make peace and the time to take a firm stand, between the glory of standing alone and the graciousness of accepting help when offered.

When they have learnt to be more true to themselves, to listen more attentively to the still, small voice within, they will be less tormented and better able to radiate forth that quality which they value above all others — peace!

As we retrace our steps, we find Agrimony to be the partner of Mustard. Mustard was for depression of an unknown cause. Agrimony is for a depression so deeply suppressed that not only is its cause unknown, the very depression itself is unrecognized and unacknowledged. Not only does the Agrimony person deceive others, they deceive themselves.

While the countenance of Mustard expresses gloom, that of

Agrimony shows forth a happy façade. Mustard's depression is overt and uncontrollable. Agrimony's is hidden and temporarily controllable by an effort of the will. Both types are endeavouring to overcome suppressed or repressed emotions.

Both need more sunshine in their life.

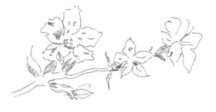

Centaury
(Centaurium erythræa)

Whereas Agrimony was a cheerful, outgoing person, whose love of peace and harmony at times induced them to surrender more ground than perhaps they need, Centaury people deliberately relinquish their own rights in the service of their family, their friends, of mankind.

In, Heal Thyself, Dr. Bach gave his understanding of the cause of disease. He spoke forcefully of the importance of each soul following its own path, without let or hindrance. This means that we must neither unduly influence, nor be unduly influenced by, another soul.

Of course, we cannot live in isolation. Caring for and helping one another is an important part of our development. Advice is one thing, domination is quite another. Trouble comes when we try to impose our will on another, or allow another to impose their will on us. Said Dr. Bach, "We must earnestly learn to develop individuality according to the dictates of our own soul, to fear no man and to see that no one interferes with, or dissuades us from, the development of our evolution." The Centaury desire to be of service so grows upon them that they become more servants than willing helpers. In their desire to express unconditional Love, they forget that Will also is a divine attribute.

This is not to say that no human soul should devote its life to the service of others. It may well be that this was the soul's intent upon incarnation, its true path in life. When this is the case, there is no error and the face of such a soul will be illumined by the glow of light from within. Contrast this with the pale, worn face of such a one who has allowed themselves to sink into a state of servitude.

Centaury people do not start out in life pale and worn. Just look at the picture of the Centaury plant. It has so many florets, as though it were trying to fill every possible space with one of its blossoms. It is only as the years go by that their Centaury good nature leads them to overspend their energy reserves. These kind and gentle people, who find it so hard to speak up for themselves, so hard to say "No", become pale, drained and worn out. The preventative approach would have us discover these people while still in the flush of their youthful enthusiasm so that their generous energy may be directed in a manner mutually beneficial to them and to society.

As the Centaury person comes to realize that their good nature is being abused, they may put on a brave face, refusing to admit to themselves, or to others, that they are finding it difficult to cope with their commitments. They may need to dip back into Agrimony, for a remedy to complement the action of the Centaury they so much need.

It is hard for the Centaury person to allow another to do something for them. The Impatiens person needed to learn to allow others slower than themselves to struggle to achieve for themselves without the interference of impatient Impatiens. Centaury must learn that others, also, need to give that they may grow spiritually and that no gift can be given without a recipient to receive. At times we best serve the highest ideal by our willingness to receive the service or gifts of others.

So many of us brought up in Christian countries were taught that the Cross represented the Self crossed out. The spiritual path was presented to us as one that required self-abnegation. We failed to treasure our 'Self', the greatest gift that God has given us.

Today there has been a shift in emphasis. We learn, rather, that we have a right to be here, as much as the trees and the stars, as the beautiful poem, Desiderata, tells us. Alas, for some the shift has been so great that it is all about 'self', but that is not the case with the Centaury person.

One would imagine that every soul which places its foot upon the spiritual path must pass through a Centaury stage, in which it learns to think of others before self, but if we are to fulfill our destiny, then our own needs must receive equal consideration. If there is justice in the Universe, surely it will ensure that each soul is guaranteed equal opportunity to develop its innate potential. Why, then, should we think that we are in some way less worthy than others?

Centaury people are good natured, kind and gentle. They do more than their fair share of work, which means that other people do less. Their generosity leads other people into selfishness.

The infant is totally self-centred. The unselfish parent denies its own needs to satisfy those of its selfish infant.

This balance has to be redressed as the child develops, for the sake of both the parent and the child. The developing child becomes aware of the competing needs of others and learns to temper its own demands. This tempering is brought about by a combination of praise and punishment. In the pursuit of the one end and in avoidance the other, the soul may become entrapped in a spiral of self-sacrifice, especially those souls whose eyes are set upon attaining eternal praise and avoiding eternal punishment. Alas, they may find the spiral a downward one.

Centaury has its place among the second nineteen remedies, the path 'home' because it does represent the 'path home' dilemma faced by the evolving soul; of developing its own individuality without interfering, or being interfered, with that of any other, of balancing the claims of its own ideals and ideas with those of its fellow travelers.

Centaury represents that part of our spiritual experience in which we yearn to empty out, to let go of all that is holding us back, hindering our progress. This is a stepping stone along the path towards our final destination.

By now you will have realized that the partner for each of the second nineteen remedies is to be found among the first nineteen in the reverse order to that in which we first studied them. Centaury finds its partner in White Chestnut and no doubt you have already seen the underlying connection between them. Both these people are slaves, the one (White Chestnut) to their own thoughts, the other (Centaury) to the thoughts, wishes and opinions of others. Each is unable to assert control over their lives. Both need to take control, to refuse to allow other influences to impinge upon them and to deflect them from their chosen path and goal. One underlying problem, two manifestations.

And so it is with all of them.

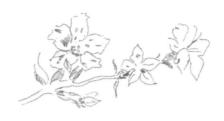

Walnut

(Juglans regia)

Walnut has two distinct spheres of action. On the one hand it provides a protecting barrier to insulate us from outside influences; on the other hand it enables us to break free from the prison in which we may have so long confined ourselves. Walnut is the remedy for those who have definite ideas and ambitions, for those who have made firm resolutions. They have passed through the Centaury stage of being easily influenced by others, or by the dictates of the body. When a person has made a decision to change, Walnut may strengthen them in their resolve. One sees the progression from the Agrimony person, with their emotional need to rely on stimulants, to the Centaury person for whom the flesh is weak no matter how willing the spirit, to the Walnut person who is now ready to make a commitment.

The Walnut people have definite ideas and ambitions but at times allow themselves to be led away from their own ideas, aims and work by the enthusiasm, convictions or strong opinions of others. No longer is the soul in the Walnut state the slave of other people's whims and wishes. It is now taking control of its life but, at times, may slip back into old habits and allow itself to be over influenced by others.

Although this remedy is made from the flowers of the Walnut tree, I feel Dr. Bach must have been guided in his choice by the knowledge that this flower is but the progenitor of the strong nut to follow. Dr. Bach spoke of this remedy giving constancy and protection from outside influences.

Chancellor states that Dr. Bach had recommended the use of this remedy for the advancing stages of life. He even quoted a number of purely physical indications for its use (teething, puberty, menopause), as well as emotional states, such as occur with changes of occupation, country, religion, and so forth.

Chancellor went on to say that Dr. Bach considered this to be the remedy for those who have resolved to take a great step forward in life, to break old conventions, to leave old limits and restrictions, to start on a new way. One feels the hope and energy as the soul has come to the realization that it serves best by fulfilling its own destiny and that that destiny is as great as the destiny of any other soul which is, has been, or ever will be.

That Dr. Bach should have mentioned change of religion, which is one of the most profound changes which any person ever undergoes, helps us to appreciate to some extent the strength and depth of the action of this remedy.

On the more physical level, probably the greatest change one experiences is the birth of one's first baby (be one male or female). Great adjustments are needed on the part of both parents, as the family dynamics will never be the same again. The birth of any subsequent children will necessitate a further negotiation of the dynamics of the expanded family; this time might not be quite so traumatic for the more experienced parents but may be very traumatic for the older child who must now share its parents' attention. And do not forget the little infant — it has made the biggest choice and change of all, incarnating once again upon this plane. The emotional change as it leaves the realm of spirit, the physical change as it breaks free from the safe confines of the womb, what greater Walnut state can there be than this?

Do not forget Walnut as life draws towards its close. When the time has come for the soul to pass over, when the resolution has been made to bid this Vale of Tears "Goodbye", then may Walnut perform its final service.

An interesting case is presented by Chancellor. We read of a spiritual healer who had become so sensitive that at times she took upon herself the physical conditions of those who came to her for healing. Walnut gave her protection from these influences and many therapists today follow her lead, taking Walnut when they feel in need of its insulating vibrations.

Although no mention is made of allergies, and we do know that we must be wary of prescribing on the basis of physical indications, yet the openness of allergy sufferers to outside influences must bring this remedy into our thoughts.

This remedy must also be considered in relation to grief. Loss of a loved one, a business, a marriage, all these bring in their wake a need for changes in outlook, changes in life patterns.

Walnut is a remedy frequently suggested when a person makes the decision to give up smoking, or to change their diet in order to lose weight. It may be a two-edged sword. If the person has been talked (or nagged) into making the change, they are being influenced by the enthusiasm, strong convictions and opinions of others. Walnut may 'protect' them from this influence and they may decide not to proceed with the change, which they did not truly desire.

This is the remedy for the new start, the new resolution — for that day which is the first day of the rest of your life! As one has spoken, so shall one perform.

Walnut is the complement of Olive. The Olive has a soft exterior but its centre is solid. The Olive person may appear soft on the outside, often committing themselves to do too much, rather like Centaury, but they have a solid centre which enables them to persist with their self-imposed tasks long after others would have given up. Walnut is the opposite.

These people may appear solid, confident, even over-confident in their ability to walk a path, even a new and challenging path, but inside they are more vulnerable than they appear. They need their firm outer shell to protect them. It must have no cracks or weaknesses. With their armour reinforced, Centaury/weak Walnut types can become strong Walnut types, able to make the necessary changes, to balance their work load, to take on only that which they are capable of performing without detriment to the self, to be strong and confident in their calling.

Walnut acts within the fifth group of remedies in a similar manner to that of Hornbeam in Group Two and Olive in Group Three. After the despondency of Gorse came the physically strengthening influence of Hornbeam; after the resignation of Wild Rose came Olive, bringing with it mental strength to regroup one's energies and move ahead. Now, following the emotionally weak state of Centaury, we find Walnut, which helps to shake off the trammels of past negative influences. It protects us from the emotional weakness which may make us doubt our own resolve in the face of other people's doubts and/or criticisms.

It was Centaury which brought the emotional strength and resolve necessary to make a change. It is Walnut which sustains that resolve. Olive brought strength to carry on along a path already chosen. Walnut brings strength to continue along the new path now selected.

Holly
(Ilex acquifolium)

All those whose cultural heritage springs from Europe will associate Holly with Christmas, the time of goodwill and happiness. This tough evergreen tree refuses to bow to the rigours of the winter chill. Its dark green leaves are quite untouched by frost and snow and its red berries bring a touch of colour to an otherwise barren landscape.

It was the flower of this plant that Dr. Bach found to contain the antidote to our negative reactions to life's vexations. The barbs of the holly leaves remind us of our reaction to the barbs of life, how often we prickle within.

Dr. Bach spoke of this remedy for thoughts of jealousy, envy, revenge or suspicion. Chancellor said hatred, envy, jealousy or suspicion. This is only a small change, but a significant one. The word 'revenge' implies an active desire to hurt another, to pay back, which is even more powerful than the 'hate' of which Chancellor speaks. This desire may not be acted out, or it may be displaced to some other person or institution, who/which may suffer in the place of the person/institution responsible for the initial internal wound. For example, a wife and/or children may suffer the bad temper of a husband who is angered by a perceived injustice at work. A gunman may shoot innocent children at school or shoppers at a shopping centre in an attempt to take revenge on some institution against which he feels powerless.

Holly is the remedy for overt hatred. It is also the remedy for those feelings of vexation which pierce our hearts from within. Dr. Bach says, "Within themselves, they may suffer much," and he completes his sentence with the comment, "often when there is no real cause for their unhappiness".

When we spoke of Walnut, we spoke of adjustments to life's changing circumstances; times of change such as puberty, marriage, childbirth, migration to a new country. So often hatred or jealousy is the legacy of our inability to adjust to changing circumstances. Remember again the child who finds that it now has to share its parents' affection with a newborn sibling — or the husband who has to share his wife's affections with their new born child! If this adjustment is not made satisfactorily, jealousy or hatred may result. Similarly, if a friend has an unexpected stroke of good fortune, a substantial lottery win, for example, and one is unable to adjust the image held to fit the changed circumstances and relationship, then jealousy may be experienced.

It has been said that forgiving one's enemies is easy compared to forgiving one's friends! Feelings of envy or jealousy towards our friends, when our conscience tells us we should be rejoicing in their good fortune, have to be expressed and wreak their havoc deep within our hearts. We may become bitter, or experience hateful feelings towards them, even though they have done nothing to hurt us. There are times when human beings do say or do things with the deliberate intention of harming someone else.

These occasions are, mercifully, few. Most of us strive to do good, if for no other reason than the selfish one of wishing to be liked.

Even in those circumstances when human justice would indicate that we have, indeed, been hard done by, Holly will help dissolve the negative energy patterns with which we are surrounding ourselves. We can surrender our grievances into the safe hands of providence, for "Vengeance is Mine, saith the Lord, I will repay". The ledger must, and will be, balanced.

When this remedy is being prepared by the boiling method, a few leaves are included along with the flowers. These are the young leaves, which have not yet grown their spikes. How true it is that the young do not prickle with hatred, envy, jealousy and suspicion, or harbor thoughts of revenge, as do older folks. Those traits develop in response to accumulated life experiences which have not been satisfactorily handled or resolved. The young child is trusting; we teach it to harbor thoughts of suspicion against fellow human beings. Alas that this should be so necessary.

It has been said that spiritual jealousy is harder to overcome than jealousy in regard to material things. Even those who have surrendered their greed for the glories of earthly success may still suffer the pangs of envy when their spiritual progress seems to them to be slow in comparison to that of some other soul. This state is more insidious but no less destructive.

Dr. Bach directed us to use either Holly or Wild Oat if a case appeared to need many remedies. "In all cases where the patient is of the active, intense type, give Holly. In patients who are of the weak, despondent type, give Wild Oat".

Has Holly no positive quality, no contribution to make to the evolution of the world? Of course it has! If we experienced no feelings of hatred or anger towards the evils and inequalities of life, how would we ever generate the energy necessary to change and overcome them? Even the Great Master took up the scourge in the Temple when he overturned the tables of the money-changers.

We must learn to hate the sin, not the sinner. If we hate the human being, instead of hating the attitude or circumstances, then the energy is misplaced and brings harm in its wake, to ourselves, if not to the other person.

How would we break out of our bonds to create a better future if this energy was not available to us? No wonder Holly follows Walnut!

The vexations for which Holly is appropriate may have their root in recent events or those of long ago and they may be of extreme or minor nature. Small irritations can fester and cause damage over time. "To irritate" can be "to anger" or "to stimulate to vital action".

These two meanings reflect the dual role of Holly. Its intense energy can be harnessed in the service of either good or evil. "Of all the trees that are in the wood, the Holly bears the crown" — so runs the old Christmas carol, and who are we to argue?

In our homeward journey we find Holly partnered by Wild Rose. Holly is the remedy for hatred and anger in its outward expression, directed against the external world. The Wild Rose resignation and apathy stem from suppressed hatred or anger, this powerful energy having been turned inwards against the self. One energy, two expressions, two remedies — two remedies which may need to be used alternately as the patient moves through the healing process.

Of the seven positive soul qualities listed by Dr. Bach, I believe Peace to be the gift of the fifth group of remedies.

Chapter Ten

For Despondency or Despair
(Group Six)

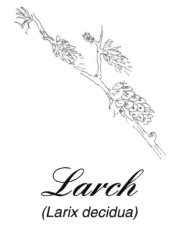

Larch
(Larix decidua)

Under the influence of Holly, we have learned not to be envious of the good fortune or abilities of others. People needing Larch have learned this lesson too well! Far from being envious, they tend to adopt an attitude of wistful admiration towards others whom they perceive as being more capable or successful than themselves.

This state of mind can afflict us at any stage of our journey. We think of the child who despairs of ever being as clever as its class mate, and so fails to make any real endeavor at school. As we proceed through life, we have brought to our attention the exploits of our fellow travelers talented in the fields of the arts, the sciences or sporting endeavours. We admire them, and rightly so. At times we are inspired to emulate them but, more frequently, we settle back into the way of thinking "I could never be like them". And that may be true in that particular aspect of life but the success of others does not define our endeavours. Each soul has a different path, different challenges to face. As life draws to a close, we may look back with satisfaction upon our achievements, forgiving ourselves that they have not been greater, on the grounds that we were not dealt a better hand.

We are even encouraged at times to take this attitude, to learn to defer to others who are held up before us as paragons of some virtue. This is a subtle way of destroying ambition and endeavour, while, at the same, appearing to encourage it. The Church builds up the saints before us as an example of holy living, but does not expect us to reach their height, for if it were attained by too many, saintliness would lose its lofty status.

This is the remedy for those who have become convinced, one way or another, that they are not as good or as capable as those around them, who expect to fail, or at least, not to excel.

Of course, we all have different talents — it would be a very boring world if this were not the case. The crucial word to note in Dr. Bach's description is 'good': "Those who do not consider themselves as good as those around them". While appreciating, without envy, the achievements of others, we must never lose sight of the fact that, in the eyes of our Creator, we have as much worth as any other soul ever created, and have as much potential.

The Larch state is not to be confused with the resigned state of Wild Rose. The Wild Rose person fails to act from apathy; the Larch person fails to act from lack of self-confidence. In some areas they may be quite content with their achievements, but something deep within them is urging them to a greater effort, even though this may not be consciously recognized.

The Larch person will often inadvertently disclose this inner aspiration to the discerning listener by reference to the achievements of others, accompanied by such statements as "I wish I could be like that/do that".

It may be that at some earlier time they have failed to achieve some goal, they may have been teased, laughed at, or scorned by some playmate — or parent. They have learned to protect themselves from recurrence of this unpleasant experience by failing to attempt anything of which they do not feel themselves easily capable.

We must not underestimate the positive qualities of Larch. To have learned genuine appreciation of others' good qualities, free of envy, jealousy, suspicion or hate, is progress indeed!

Imitation is the sincerest form of flattery and any 'super-star' worthy of that title would be more delighted with the fan who worked hard to emulate them than they would be with applause from the side-lines. The uncritical admiration which the devotee expresses towards its idol, be that idol human or divine, is but a faint reflection of the devotion which we will one day be capable of expressing. No true teacher, or guru, is satisfied with a student or pupil who merely admires them. They do not look for passive admiration; they look for sustained effort. At times we may feel like the page-boy on the Feast of Stephen. Bidden by his master to bring the flesh, the wine and the pine logs hither, so that the poor man might dine that Christmas tide, he looked at the elements he would have to battle to perform this worthy task and felt inadequate. He hesitated to set out for fear that he would be unable to complete the journey. However, he heeded the words of his saintly king, Wenceslas:

> "Mark my footsteps, good my page,
> Tread thou in them boldly.
> Thou shalt find the winter's rage
> Freeze they blood less coldly."

And so he set out, finding that he could accomplish more than he had believed.

We need to grow through the stage of Larch, so that we may once more fix our gaze firmly upon the mountain top, so that we may answer the challenge to venture where we have never ventured before.

Larch finds itself partnered by Honeysuckle. We recall that Honeysuckle was the remedy for unproductive wishful thinking — looking back and wishing that things had turned out differently or that we could recapture some past triumph or achievement. Neither Honeysuckle nor Larch expect, or strive for change. The underlying issue is perception of self-worth, past, present and future.

Honeysuckle may wish to rest on the laurels of its past achievements, failing to realize that no matter how great they may have been, they are past. It is the future which counts and how we build upon the foundation we have laid. Larch is not so backward looking, and this is progress, but they are still hesitating to push forward, to strive to achieve goals not within easy reach.

So often, the lack of self-confidence we feel today can be traced back to incidents which happened in our past, even as far back as our childhood. We carry forward into the present the negative evaluations of the past — unable to let them go. Honeysuckle and Larch march hand in hand.

Clematis also covered wishful thinking, but inasmuch as it was forward thinking, the dreamer was anticipating/planning change. In fact, the Clematis person may well over-estimate their abilities — quite the opposite of Larch.

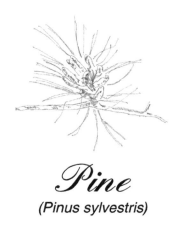

Pine
(Pinus sylvestris)

The beautiful pine tree provides the next of our remedies and is for the state of self-blame. "Even when successful they think they could have done better and they are never content with their effort or results."

The Larch people failed to attempt in expectation of failure. Pine people attempt, but fail in their own estimation. The Larch state of passive wistfulness has given way to the Pine state of active endeavor, but there is no satisfaction. The Pine people set themselves a high standard and judge themselves harshly when they fail, as fail they sometimes must. I spoke earlier of how much easier it is to forgive an enemy than a friend. Hardest of all is it to forgive oneself!

Of course, there are some people who fail to take

responsibility for their actions, who blame others for all that goes wrong. (We will meet their remedy shortly.) But all people experience guilt at some time and it can be one of the most destructive emotions with which we ever have to deal.

One of the advantages of using the Bach Flower remedies is that we do not need to make an evaluation of rightness or wrongness. It may be that the person does have a good reason to feel guilty; it may be that they are condemning themselves quite unnecessarily. It matters not; it is the attitude of mind that must guide us to the remedy's use.

If we cannot learn from our mistakes, we are condemned to repeat them. But once the lesson is learnt, the experience should be released. If we try to limp through life dragging behind us the chain of past events, we will be slow indeed to make any progress.

Dr. Bach was harsh in his attitude towards sufferers from self-blame. He spoke of these people attaching faults to themselves and of claiming responsibility even for the faults of others. He saw it as a form of self-centredness that we should consider ourselves so important and powerful that our actions should have so profound an effect on other people.

At times they do, and at times those effects may even be devastating. If there is any way in which the wrong can be redressed, then we should act at the first opportunity. If there is not, torturing ourselves with feelings of guilt will be of benefit to no one.

"If only I could" has been replaced with "If only I had" or 'had not", as the case may be.

Between incarnations, we sleep the sleep of forgetfulness. If, during each incarnation, we were to be burdened by conscious remembrance of our past mistakes, we would be so overcome with shame that we would be reluctant to face the world at all. We are blest by having these memories withheld from us, although the cumulative effect of these experiences, which has given us our present character, stays with us. We need to take heed of this lesson and to apply it in our daily lives.

Said Dr. Bach, "Let us not give a moment's regret to the slips by the way. No great ascent was ever made without faults and falls and they must be regarded as experiences which will help us to stumble less in the future. No thoughts of past errors must ever depress us; they are over and finished, and the knowledge thus gained will help us avoid a repetition of them. Yesterday's mistake is the basis for tomorrow's achievement."

"If only" — the two saddest words in the English language!

There are other forms of guilt, some of them suffered more prominently by those endeavouring to follow the spiritual path. There may be guilt about accepting money, even for services rendered, feeling that help to one's fellow travelers should be 'freely given' even by those who have made the healing therapies their life's work. Once Dr. Bach abandoned orthodox medicine and started prescribing only his flower remedies, he charged no fee, but Dr. Bach had enough savings to support his simple life style, although he did accept gifts from close friends towards his maintenance. I would presume here to question Dr. Bach's decision. Although noble, should not the recipient of the help be allowed to recompense their helper in some way? A small contribution from such persons as were able to make it might have been appropriate.

I support Dr. Bach's decision not to charge the large fee often associated with medical treatment, but an appropriate remuneration would seem to me to be beneficial for both parties. It is the love of money which is the root of all evil, not money itself which is — or should be — but a measure of an exchange of energies. Poverty is not a necessary prerequisite to holiness.

Some people feel guilty about taking time off work, as if their work were so important some calamity would ensue if they did not labour. This is a manifestation of false pride. (We will meet their remedy shortly, too.)

Unfortunately, guilt makes life a living hell. How appropriate that Pine should be the tree that graces our homes at Christmas time. Beneath its sweet smelling branches, we place our gifts of friendship. In silent vigil, it watches over us at this time as we forgive past hurts and extend the hand of friendship to those who may have wronged us. As the Yule-tide log burns brightly in the hearth, we feel its flames purifying us of the dross we have accumulated during the year. Its fragrance wafts through our home, bringing its cleansing aroma to every nook and cranny. Its task has been completed when we have extended forgiveness, not only to others, but to ourselves.

As we learned with Holly to surrender to Providence the task of addressing any wrong we may have suffered at the hands of others, so with Pine we must learn the harder lesson of surrendering to Providence whatever balancing of the books it may decree with regard to our own activities. We must not take it upon ourselves to punish ourselves; that will be done in the most appropriate manner and at the most perfect time, by a wisdom that is greater than ours.

It would be wrong to think that the Pine state has no positive benefit, for without an appreciation of wrong-doing, without a feeling of guilt, we would have no conscience, no guide to point the way to perfection. The infant has no conscience to direct its behaviour. It acts in accordance with its instincts and desires. It cannot choose to do right until it has learned that which is wrong.

Through guilt we grow.

Pine represents both a passing mood and a long-term state of mind. All of us feel guilt in some degree or another at some time or another but there are some people who pass through life in a continuous state of self-blame, appropriating to themselves guilt for life circumstances, not all of which are under their control. The parent of the delinquent or criminal may say, "If only I had been able to work and had money to buy things, my child might not have thought it necessary to steal". In fact, there are countless numbers of children of working parents, of non-working parents, of broken homes, of stable homes, of loving parents, of violent parents, who do not go astray. In the final analysis, each child is responsible for its own actions, yet how often the parent claims the responsibility.

The link connecting Pine with its partner Clematis is that of responsibility.

In the Clematis state, the soul fails to take upon itself the degree of responsibility appropriate for its stage of development, drifting through life in a cloud of good intentions, excusing any shortfall in result by saying, "I meant well". Alas, the path to hell is paved with good intentions! Pine is quite the reverse. It accepts the burden of guilt, not only for its own actions, but also for the actions of others, and finds this path also leads to a living hell. These people refuse to accept that it is not humanly possible to foresee all possible circumstances, all possible results of their actions, all eventualities and that "It seemed like a good idea at the time" is sufficient justification for sincere and honest effort.

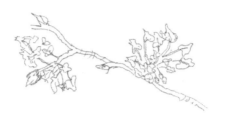

Elm
(Ulmus procera)

Responsibility is an ongoing theme in our study of Elm. The soul is firmly established, having a clear idea of the path that it wishes to follow. These people are doing good work, often for the benefit of humanity. They hope to achieve something of importance and are, therefore, willing to shoulder responsibility, without being burdened down by guilt.

Like Pine before them, they have a tendency to take on too much. They are capable people and others learn to rely on them and, like Centaury, they hate to let people down. In many ways they resemble Centaury, the chief point of difference being that Elm is not being imposed upon by others. The tasks they take on are of their own choosing and are usually for the benefit of others less fortunate than themselves. They are frequently to be found in positions of responsibility and trust: teachers, doctors, nurses, priests, healers, social workers. They are in positions where it will affect many others if they fall sick or take a holiday. No one is indispensable, but the Elm type comes as close to this as anybody.

Is it any wonder that at times they feel inadequate for their self-appointed task? Unlike Larch, who hesitated to try, Elm tries too hard.

As Pine before them, they strive for perfection, but they are more forgiving of their own shortcomings. They understand that even executives can make mistakes at times. They learn from their mistakes. Turning stumbling blocks into stepping stones, they resolve to work harder and do better in future.

Dr. Bach tells us that there come times when the Elm soul feels that it has taken on too heavy a burden: "That the task they have undertaken is too difficult and not within the power of a human being." The Elm person is not the type to give up. We have left our suicidal remedies behind — there are no more ahead that consider this option. Elm people will work until they drop, and sometimes they do.

Because these people are so competent, others do not realize how exhausted they are. While Elm is their 'type' remedy, they may well benefit from the remedy of another tree we studied previously, Olive, because they do indeed become exhausted in body and mind.

Whereas Larch people experience ongoing lack of self-confidence and Pine people experience ongoing guilt, Elm experiences both of these states only temporarily, and frequently together: lack of confidence that they will be able to continue and guilt that they may find it necessary to ask for help.

Elm finds its partner in Wild Oat. Wild Oat people had a feeling of purpose, even ambition, but were still searching for their path in life. They represented unfulfilled potential. Elm people have found their path, they are aware of their mission in life.

Potential is being fulfilled.

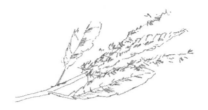

Sweet Chestnut

(Castanea sativa)

This is the last of the four remedies which Dr. Bach chose from the family of the Chestnut. It is not a 'type' remedy, being rather for a state, a state which Dr. Bach says happens "to some people". This is the only remedy for which Dr. Bach makes this qualification.

It is easy to see why Sweet Chestnut follows Elm because it is the remedy for those times when the mind or body feels as if it had borne to the utmost limits of its endurance and now it must give way. We spoke of the fact that Elm people push themselves to their limit, refusing to give in, to take a rest, until they reach the point of exhaustion. If they fail to accept the help offered by Hornbeam and Olive, when indicated, they may find themselves in need of Sweet Chestnut.

The Sweet Chestnut state of distress seems to challenge the very belief in all that is right and good. "I have worked so hard, always tried to do that which is right, why do I suffer so?" It is the cry of Job, the saint undergoing the tribulations of the spiritual path. It is the long, dark night of the soul, that time of truth when one is brought face to face with the meaning of reality.

Lest I seem to be exaggerating, read again Dr. Bach's words. He spoke of an anguish so great as to seem unbearable. "It seems that there is nothing but destruction and annihilation left to face." Chancellor quotes Dr. Bach as saying it was for that "appalling despair when it seems the very soul itself is suffering destruction".

Dr. Bach promised a remedy for every negative state to which mankind is subject and history bears witness to the depths of despair which some may be called upon to suffer.

As Hornbeam was to physical stress, Olive to mental stress, Walnut to emotional stress, so Sweet Chestnut is to spiritual stress.

The state described seems to be so profound that one may feel that "it won't happen to me" or to anyone else living in civilized suburbia. Surely only those suffering the torments of war, of famine, of torture, or enduring the privations of concentration camps could be brought to so profound and poignant a state? Not so!

Working in the healing professions, I have been amazed at how many tell of having passed through Sweet Chestnut states, usually without anyone else being aware of the depth of their suffering. Many have been Elm type personalities. Because it is not within the nature of the Elm person to give in, to complain, they continue to perform their duties to the best of their ability, while feeling estranged from normality, as if in a daze. The state is described as being one of utter emptiness, a total void. One has given one's all and there is nothing left. It is as though the Chalice of Life has been drained. One feels totally alone, even in the midst of friends.

I can do no better than to quote once more from Chancellor: "a world where sight is not seeing and sound is not hearing, where the closest person is millions of miles away". And again: "I feel I am no longer worthy even to pray. I am a complete void. I am so alone".

While Sweet Chestnut states usually develop over a time of prolonged stress, Sweet Chestnut must not be forgotten for profound grief. Whether the grief be for permanent loss through death or partial loss through a broken relationship, the feeling of utter devastation and desolation which occurs for some people at these times is covered well by Sweet Chestnut.

These people do not contemplate suicide. It is not in their nature, yet they yearn for Fate to relieve them of their responsibilities by granting them the blessing of eternal sleep. Exhausting human resources, the soul finally sends out a call for help which is heard in the realms beyond.

Since all souls were created equal, and all must share equal experience, all must pass through the Sweet Chestnut state at some point in their evolution but not necessarily every incarnation. As with all states covered by these thirty-eight remedies, the same state can be experienced at a number of levels, much like octaves on the musical scale. The Sweet Chestnut state will be more profound the greater the level of spiritual evolution and the further the progress along the path.

This may well be the greatest remedy of all.

We look back and see Sweet Chestnut partnered by Hornbeam. Both are remedies for those who feel they have not sufficient strength to bear the burden life has placed upon them. The Hornbeam state is similar to, but not as profound as, that of Sweet Chestnut.

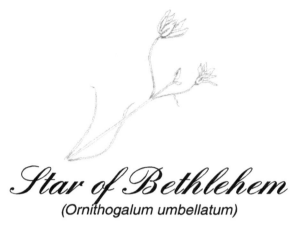

Star of Bethlehem
(Ornithogalum umbellatum)

Star of Bethlehem is a common weed in many parts of England and Scotland and was given its name because it is found abundantly in Palestine where its bulbs are cooked and eaten.

Whenever one experiences shock, Star of Bethlehem is needed. It is not used as much as it might be because it is often replaced by Rescue Remedy, of which it is an ingredient. Star of Bethlehem is the remedy for those in great distress, whether this be the result of bad news, accident, fright or sudden illness.

This is a major remedy for grief. Dr. Bach said "For those who for a time refuse to be consoled". In the early stages of grief, the griever does not want to be consoled, to be told, "Never mind. You will (soon) feel better. Time will heal". For a while, they feel the need to wallow in their grief, to experience it to the full until, being satisfied, the desire fades.

Speaking of grief, let us not forget this remedy for the infant after its "shocking" birth experience. Even if the birth is not especially traumatic by human standards, the grief of leaving behind the astral plane, coupled with the shock of finding oneself back here, once again, (and with you as a parent!) surely calls for the soothing calmness this flower can bring. If we can but pacify the influence of these first few hours or days, we may do much to assist the soul to form a beautiful relationship with its surrounding world.

Star of Bethlehem should also be considered for those whose contact with the other planes is not always pleasant. I speak of bad dreams or nightmares. While Rock Rose is indicated for the great fear of nightmares, Star of Bethlehem may be needed if the dream leaves a residual sense of having been traumatized. On waking, the fear has dissipated, but the unpleasant memory lingers one.

Star of Bethlehem, this flower from the Holy Land, should also be considered for any person who has, or has had in the past, some involvement with the darker arts, known as Black Magic.

While Rescue Remedy is appropriately used for short term emergency situations, Star of Bethlehem may be needed over more extended periods. Conditions of distress or unhappiness are, alas, not always brief, as we discovered to our cost in our Sweet Chestnut state.

We have noticed how the remedies of hope and survival always follow those of despair and we are not let down. The greatest despair remedy is aided in its healing by the strongest and most profound of the revivifiers.

Experience has shown that Star of Bethlehem can help heal the scars of past trauma, even though these were occasioned many years previously. Increasingly the medical profession is investigating the connection between emotional states and the onset of disease. It is advisable to give Star of Bethlehem to the person who has a history of emotional trauma as it is not always easy to recognize the indications of past sufferings, unless they are very severe.

Even if the person insists that they are "over it now", a precautionary prescription of Star of Bethlehem would not be out of place. It can do no harm.

Looking back at the earlier Group 2 remedies, we realize that the discouragement suffered by Gentian, Gorse and Hornbeam people related very much to the affairs of everyday living. The emotional states being suffered by those for whom the current group of remedies is needed are of a different kind, touching a far deeper level, although foreshadowed by their earlier counterparts.

Gorse had given up belief that anything more could be done for them. They held "so little hope of relief". Star of Bethlehem is also experiencing great unhappiness, refusing to be consoled because they, too, see little hope of relief, of future joy. Star of Bethlehem has its deeper action because if follows a greater depth of experience. Gorse hoped for peace through change in external circumstances; its partner, Star of Bethlehem, has realized that true peace comes only from within the self.

As with groups two and three, so also it is with groups five and six. The first group of the pair relates to more concrete experiences, the second to more immaterial experiences.

Dr. Bach worked strenuously during his last two years of life to discover remedies which he knew would be necessary for these more profound states. Of the eight remedies in this group, none belong to the original Twelve Healers. Oak, alone, is one of the Four Helpers. The remaining seven are from the final group of nineteen; all are trees, six trees of substantial size and strength.

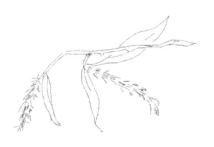

Willow
(Salix vitellina)

Although the Willow selected by Dr. Bach is not the Weeping Willow which so commonly graces the riverbanks of England, it is the same family. The graceful Weeping Willow, whose delicate bows droop downwards towards the waters running beneath its shade, has long

been the symbol of heartbreak. It was the custom in Elizabethan times for spurned suitors to wear a spray of Willow on their shoulder to proclaim their rejection — although one wonders how heart-broken they really were! Nevertheless, "to wear the willow" is an expression still to be found in the English language.

The leaves of the Willow were supposed to resemble tear-drops, the tree's affinity to water lending added weight to this supposed resemblance. Dr. Bach found the flowers of its close relative, the salix vitellina, to be the remedy for those who had suffered adversity or misfortune, find these difficult to accept without complaint or resentment, so maybe the young bucks of yesteryear were not so far out in their selection!

The slender branches of the Willow teach us that it is better to bend with the storm than try to resist. Storms are part of life, and while we will inevitably be tossed about by their powerful currents, if we are pliable in our attitude, we may rapidly settle back again once the storm is passed. Failure to adjust to the setbacks and disheartenments of life burdens us with resentment and hinders our progress.

Willow is known as the remedy for bitterness, and with good cause, for Dr. Bach tells us that these people feel that they have not deserved so great a trial, that it is unjust, and that they become embittered. This is a salutary lesson to us. Having just considered the trials of the Sweet Chestnut state, let us not be deceived into thinking that all come through with flying colours. An examination which all students automatically pass is not worthy of the name. Some may feel bitter temporarily as they work at soothing their ruffled feathers. Others may find it more difficult to be forgiving of life. No wonder we require so many incarnations to reach perfection.

The Willow person is opposite to Pine. Whereas Pine took an undeserved blame, Willow off-loads blame for its own failings or actions on to others or life circumstances.

At times it may be difficult to distinguish between the anger of Holly and the bitterness of Willow. One is directed outwards, the other inwards, but the ever-restless ebb and flow of emotions almost guarantees that both will be needed at some time. Dr. Bach helps us to distinguish the one state from the other by explaining that the Willow person tends to become more introverted than they previously were. "They often take less interest and are less active in those things of life which they had previously enjoyed." It is as though some of the spirit has gone out of them.

Children are more open to expressing their grievances and also more quick to overcome them. As we pass through life, we expect positive experiences to outweigh the negative, to be able to look back with satisfaction on a job well done. Not always is this the case (from a human point of view) despite our best endeavours. Life may deal us a cruel blow and all that we have worked for may seem lost to us. With not much earthly time left to regroup and recoup, it is only too easy to lapse into bitterness at perceived injustices. We see, then, that Willow is a remedy frequently indicated in life's later stages.

One example of a situation in which Willow may be required at a younger age is that of a child born with a disability or a person disabled by accident or illness. It is understandable that these people should feel bitter at times, although one must not assume that they do. Many people with disabilities are remarkably cheerful, putting able-bodied people to shame. Often it is the parent/family which is more bitter.

It would be wrong to assume that Willow is only appropriate for people who present as whingers or complainers. In practice I have found it an extremely valuable remedy for many delightful patients, who have repressed their feelings of bitterness because they believed that those who held such thoughts were unworthy. Only by listening carefully to their story was one able to detect that some incident, mentioned apparently only in passing, still rankled within their heart.

Not one of us passes through life without suffering what seem to us to be injustices and endeavouring to follow the Light does not guarantee us immunity from resentment. The fact that this remedy appears so late among the thirty-eight tells us something about the state of soul development to which it is appropriate and for which it brings sweet relief.

Dr. Bach gave us the clue to the overcoming of this stage when he told us that the Willow person often judges life much by the success which it brings. So long as we cling to the notion that worldly achievements are the standards against which we are to be measured, so long will we be tempted to judge ourselves by comparison with our fellow travelers. Reading that "all things work together for them that fear God" is one thing; practicing this belief in daily life is quite another. "They feel that they have not deserved so great a trial".

Even saints ask, "Why me?" at times — or even simply "Why?"

Willow's partner is Gentian. We recall that Gentian was the remedy for those who were discouraged by setbacks in the affairs of their daily life. Under Willow, this discouragement has become deeper, has grown to bitterness and resentment. It is not always easy to accept that the trials and tribulations of everyday living are those by which we grow spiritually. We do not need to undergo some arcane experience in the darkest depths of some ancient pyramid in order to pass another step forward along the spiritual path. The earth plane is our school; It provides enough lessons for us all, right here, at home.

In Willow we have a similar emotion to that of Gentian, but it is experienced with a deeper degree of intensity. The doubt of Gentian is a doubt of self in response to small delays or hindrances in life. The doubt of Willow is a doubt in the justice of the Universe which develops in response to greater trials and tribulations.

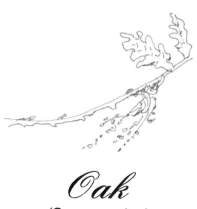

Oak
(Quercus robur)

The great English Oak — sacred tree of the Druids — whose strong branches, so legend says, gave shelter to the fugitive Prince Charles fleeing from Cromwell's troops, ensuring him the opportunity to live to fight another day and later to claim his rightful crown as Charles II.

Heart of Oak — the very words bespeak strength and the ability to battle against all odds.

Dr. Bach found this remedy to be the remedy for those who struggle and fight strongly, either when they are sick or in connection with the affairs of their daily life. Perseverance is their watchword. They will try again and again, even though things may seem hopeless.

Down, but not out, these people know that there is only one way to go and that is up. When life deals a tough hand, what is to be done? Basically, whinge or get on. Some people are able to by-pass or suppress the whinging stage; others feel the need to make known their displeasure (Willow) but in the final analysis this achieves nothing, apart from a few sympathetic grunts from our long suffering friends.

While we do receive help from others in our hour of need (because most people are kind and helpful), others cannot solve our problems. Hour after hour, day after day, year after year, life time after life time, in the end it is up to us. If we do not overcome obstacles this time, then we will have to do so next, so we might as well put the past behind us and battle on.

Following severe setbacks, especially those which appear unjust, Willow will tend to lose heart, to take less interest in those things at which they had previously worked. Oak people have a greater inborn strength which enables them to pick up the pieces and start afresh again.

Because of their inherent strength of will and basic reliability, others tend to lay their burdens upon them, but the Oak people have broad shoulders and usually they can bear it. Described as the backbone of society, they can be depended upon to honour their commitments.

There is no indecision with Oak. Once determined upon a course of action, they will pursue it, unless, and until, they prove to themselves that it is unproductive and another direction needs to be taken. They are steady workers, performing their duties in whatever situation of life it has pleased God to call them. They are less interested in fame, or power, or money than they are in a job well done.

The Oak people are quieter in doing their good work than the Elms. The Elms set out to do good in the world, and tend to hold positions of prominence which afford them recognition, whether consciously sought or not. Oak has realized that they also serve who only stand and wait. They are more content to do good wherever they are found, realizing the truth of the words of the Great Master "Inasmuch as ye do it unto the least of these little ones, ye do it unto me".

I spoke of the breakdown which an Elm person might suffer. This is not the same as the state of exhaustion which an Oak person may experience if they persistently overwork. Oak are secure in their beliefs and do not suffer the torments of doubt about Truth and the Purpose of Life that might Elm. Under extreme stress, Elm may suffer a spiritual crisis. No matter what storms and tempests may be raging about them, the Oak people have an inner strength which stems from a perfect belief that God is in his heaven and that all is right with the world no matter how inscrutable his way may appear to the eye of mortal Man.

They are practical people, full of common sense, who take the attitude "Who are we to question the wisdom of providence?" They have learnt to apply themselves to the problem in hand and to leave the evils of tomorrow (and of yesterday) to take care of themselves.

Oak is the higher vibration of Scleranthus. The Scleranthus person had recognized the need to make their own decisions, rather than rely on the advice of others (Cerato) and were developing the ability to fight their own battles. However, they still had difficulty with decision making, and the state of indecision tended to dissipate their energies, energies which they should have been directing towards the task in hand. Oak has now won those battles. They no longer suffer from indecision. They direct their energies into the most practical path and achieve results through sheer perseverance.

Their vision set firmly on their final goal, with Sir Galahad they are able to say, "My strength is as the strength of ten, because my heart is pure".

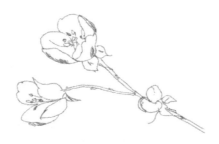

Crab Apple
(Malus sylvestris)

Bitter may be its fruit, but beautiful is its blossom.

This remedy is unique among those of which Dr. Bach wrote inasmuch as that he gave an indication for its external use as well as for its internal. Dr. Bach described this flower as the remedy of cleansing and his indications are very interesting.

As an external cleanser for wounds, Dr. Bach said that it purifies wounds if the patient has reason to believe that some poison has entered which must be drawn out. This is a rather elaborate and quaint method of expressing his message. Why did he not simply say that it purified wounds? Does it purify only if the patient believes poison has entered? And why 'poison', not 'bacteria'?

The Crab Apple people feel that there is something about themselves which is not quite clean (or perfect). This imperfection may be physical or it may relate to an emotional situation, but, whatever it is, it fills their field of vision, blotting out other more important matters. At times it may be displaced onto another person, their perceived fault consuming the Crab Apple person's attention. For example, the partner who smokes — the Crab Apple person feeling unclean because they are forced to breathe the same polluted air. Crab Apple may use "You'll develop lung cancer" as a stick with which to beat the unfortunate partner into submission, but their true fear is that they will suffer through their contact with the transgressor. Being close to the smoker, the drinker, the scruffy child, makes them feel unclean.

It must not be thought that all Crab Apple people are against smoking. Some may smoke quite happily, but be worried about a pimple or wart which they feel mars their perfection.

Crab Apple should not be given routinely to people with skin disorders just because these make the therapist feel unclean. It is true that many such people do feel unclean and Crab Apple may be appropriate, if the thought of a single pimple fills them with horror.

Crab Apple may help in letting go of some undesirable habit, such as smoking or drinking, but only if the person regards the habit as unclean in some way. The therapist must be careful not to impose their own view upon the patient, or assume that the patient feels the same way that they do.

We remember that the Oak person demonstrated singleness of mind. With the Crab Apple person this has been converted into rigidity of mind, fixation of thought. Once an idea or thought becomes entrenched, they will not, or cannot, let it go. The fixation may be about something quite trivial. Indeed, Dr. Bach goes out of his way to make this quite clear by saying, "There may be more serious disease which is almost disregarded compared to the one thing upon which they concentrate".

These thoughts are quite different from those of White

Chestnut, which are random thoughts, usually related to the business of the day, which go round and round in the mind. The Crab Apple thoughts are specific and usually relate to matters of cleanliness or purity. The offending thoughts may relate to something which was said by them, or to them, later regretted. This instance cannot be forgotten. If it was something unkind or untrue, the thought of it will torment them, even if the event occurred a long time ago.

This state bears some resemblance to Pine, with its feeling of guilt, but there is a subtle difference. Pine relates to some occurrence or circumstance. Crab Apple relates to the self. It is not the event which is regretted, but being, not of having done something which was substandard, but of being substandard. Pine is likely to have difficulty letting go of something they said or did to someone else. Crab Apple is more likely to have difficulty letting go of something someone else said or did to them.

On one level, Crab Apple relates very much to the psychological disorder known as obsessive or obsessive compulsive. This disorder relates to fixed thoughts or thoughts which cause compulsive actions, usually related to hand-washing, cleaning, avoiding contamination in some way.

Crab Apple finds its partner in Cerato. Whereas the Cerato person constantly sought advice, lacked self-direction and readily absorbed impressions from others, Crab Apple people are fixed in their ideas and find it difficult to change, even when they want to. With both remedies the issue is one of discrimination, sorting out the good from the bad, the wheat from the chaff. With Cerato, the issues relate to everyday affairs, what is the right thing to do; with Crab Apple the issue relates to perception of self — what is the right thing to be?

As we have travelled through the sixth group of remedies, you will have noticed not only that they relate to more intense states than did the earlier remedies, but that they relate more to states of being than states of doing.

The gift for the sixth group of remedies is the healing quality of Hope. With hope and anticipation let us move on now to the seventh and last group.

Chapter Eleven

Over-care for the Welfare of Others
(Group Seven)

Chicory
(Chicorium intybus)

Speaking of the glorious blue of the Chicory flowers, Dr. Bach remarked that it seemed to him to be the nearest earthly colour to that one associated with Our Lady and it is indeed a most beautiful flower to begin our last group.

Looking at this plant, one cannot but be struck by the unusual placement of its bloom. The flower springs from the centre of the stem, only one flower being fully open at one time. This illustrates to us that we are still dealing with remedies for self-centredness. We have now passed from the need only for personal perfection, as evinced by Crab

Apple, to the need for perfection in one's family or close personal circle. Chicory realizes that solitary perfection is as satisfactory as living alone in a glass house — without others to share, it is an empty experience.

The over-care of Chicory must not be confused with the over-concern experienced by Red Chestnut. The Red Chestnut concerns stem from fear, fear of how they will cope if the loved one is injured or killed, fear of what others will say if they appear to have been careless. Chicory does not suffer from these fears because these people have complete confidence in their own abilities, so much so that they think they know better than anyone else what is best. Chicory is interested in the welfare of their family, of their immediate circle, not in that of humanity at large. Of course, they will have the usual concern that does anyone concerning political situations, the environment and other major issues, but these will not call forth the fiercely protective instincts which are so prominent in Chicory with regard to their immediate circle.

Like Crab Apple, Chicory will be slow to forget an insult, either against themselves or their family. However, they can put the matter aside at will until the appropriate time comes for them to recall it, and settle the score as only Chicory knows how. Chicory are basically strong people; they feel quite competent to take on the responsibility of caring for all members of their family, any close friends, stray relatives, and, possibly, stray animals, if the need should arise.

Chicory is the matriarch of the family. Like the mother hen, fiercely defensive of any of her brood who may be under attack, she is continually fussing over those lower than her in the pecking order. They must be brought into line and made to understand their role in life, which is preserving that which the Chicory person has spent so much effort attaining.

One must not forget that children can be Chicory too. Many a parent is bossed around by its offspring. Anyone who believes that one or two sharp smacks will bring any child into line has never tried to rear a baby Chicory! I have found it quite an effective remedy for babies who wake several times during the night, not because they are hungry, but because they want attention. Think of it for the child who kicks and screams whenever being left with the unfortunate baby-sitter. Once the parent has left, Chicory children may be all sweetness and light as they charm the baby-sitter into spoiling them, letting them stay up late, reading them stories and generally lavishing attention upon them. And attention Chicory wants. Woe betide anyone who tries to bloom at the same time as they!

Chicory is well aware of the strength of the mind. They learnt young that the might of father's arm was small when compared with the might of Chicory's will. They will rarely resort to physical means to impose their will At times they may even pretend to be weak in order to gain an emotional advantage, especially as they grow older and want to keep their off-spring near them.

Illness and old age may be used as reasons why the newly married son or daughter should bring the new spouse back to the family home to live rather than acquire a place of their own, even though the older Chicory might be quite capable of managing alone. Before the wedding,

Chicory are more concerned with how much they will miss their off-spring, how empty the house will seem, than they are with the future happiness of the young couple. They may even (secretly) hope that the marriage will fail so that the fledgling will return to the nest.

To Chicory, the greatest achievement in life is a grown, and growing, family, and, if move out the children must, then let them buy houses nearby so that the circle of influence may be extended. These are the parents who oppose a marriage but come around once grandchildren arrive. Christmas would not be complete if they were not all around the dining table. That the other in-laws may have equal claim is scarcely considered.

We all know the reputation, just or unjust, of the Prima Donna acting in a Chicory manner towards her long-suffering directors and managers, throwing temper tantrums when these are likely to bring rewards. These stage-managed performances are reputed to be short-lived, the tears drying quickly enough when there is no audience to fascinate. If the star and the director both are Chicory — pity the rest of the cast — although they may understand each other well.

Similarly, in a family there may be a parent and child who are both Chicory. The relationship is likely to be stormy and unpleasant for other members of the family, although the two Chicories may have a strong bond between them.

Is there, then, no positive side to Chicory? Is it so wrong to desire that those whom one loves be near one?

Look again at the Chicory flower. We noted its beautiful colour, its central position, its outwardly radiating petals. But what holds these petals in place? A central point to which they are all attached. We may think of the petals as radiating outwards, or as being firmly centred.

The sun radiates outwards its light and its warmth and for centuries has been used as an analogy for Divine Love. But the sun also has a powerful gravitational pull. Were this not so, the Earth and the other planets of the solar system would be flung even further into the outer realms of the Universe. We owe our lives on this Earth to this inward pull of the Sun as much as we do to its outwardly radiating heat and light. The Universe demands a balance between the two forces, outgoing and in-drawing.

Is it not possible that during our evolutionary development we have need to experience an ell-encompassing selfish love as well as unselfish love? We speak often of the unselfish love of God but does not even God's love have its selfish side? Is there anything more Chicory than the love Divine Mother lavishes upon her children, drawing them ever closer to her heart, watching over every action and correcting every fault?

When Chicory blooms in the fullness of its perfection, it expresses love balanced by wisdom. In giving, with no thought of receiving, the love of the Chicory mother, human or Divine, draws her children to her, not from duty, or compulsion, but because they delight in being in the presence of one who is both loving and loved, without reservation.

When speaking of the Chicory person, Dr. Bach said that they enjoy correcting that which they consider wrong. This 'enjoyment' may be purely selfish but it may also reflect unselfish pleasure in the development of human potential. As with all emotions, it is not the emotion itself which is good or evil, but its manifestation. The role of Chicory, as of its partner, Red Chestnut, before it is to transmute, 'Smother love,' into 'Mother love'. These two remedies assist our relationship with our relations.

Chicory leads us from self-centredness to Self-Centredness.

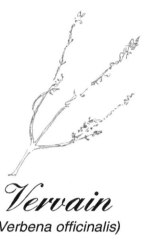

Vervain
(Verbena officinalis)

Whether Vervain reminds one of the three-pronged fork of the Devil goading his hapless victims in the nether-regions of Hell, the trident of Neptune as he rules his watery kingdom below, or of Britannia as she triumphantly rules the waves above, Vervain portrays a powerful symbol or, perhaps one should say, a symbol of power.

With Vervain we move away from our concern with our immediate family to a wider concern with the human family. The Chicory (and Crab Apple) fixed ideas and principles are still in evidence but Vervain looks to include far more people within the scope of its caring.

Vervain shows us that human aspirations reach upward in different directions, that there is room for all to branch out. When each respects the individuality of the other, all may flourish.

Vervain people have great enthusiasm for their daily work, forging straight ahead and rarely changing the direction of their thoughts and ideas. They wish others to share their enthusiasm, their success. In this they are not selfish. They are hard-working and may suffer ill health as a result of their refusal to rest. While Elm continued to work from a sense of duty (how will others manage without me?), Vervain continues to work through enthusiasm for their task. Like Elm, their project may be directed towards some good cause, or it may be a venture of a more commercial nature, it matters not. They love their work, and want to be surrounded by other people with as much energy and enthusiasm as themselves.

Whereas the Impatiens people were inclined to say, "Leave it to me. I will get the job done more quickly on my own," Vervain tends towards the attitude, "If I can do it, so can you," and they are quite happy to allow others to help. Indeed, they both expect and appreciate teamwork.

Vervain is sometimes referred to as the 'Missionary's remedy" because Dr. Bach used the words "wish to convert all around them," but there are many ideas and attitudes, other than religious, which we may wish others to share. We may even wish to convert our neighbour to our favourite brand of soap powder! It is the attitude of mind which is important, not its field of action.

We see how closely Vervain follows the Chicory state of mind. Chicory also believed they knew best but were more close-minded in directing their energies towards perfecting their immediate world (family and friends). Vervain is expansive in outlook. They have the energy and enthusiasm which makes them feel up to tackling anything — anywhere in the world, if necessary. However, this delight In their work can inspire the Vervain who never leaves their village as much as he who reaches for the stars.

Dr. Bach tells us that these people have strong wills and much courage when convinced they are right. These are people who will face any odds to bring about a reform which they feel is much needed. The flame of their enthusiasm burns more brightly than any martyr's fire.

One of Vervain's most attractive qualities is loyalty. There is no other remedy which manifests this quality so enthusiastically. While Oak will doggedly keep on keeping on, Vervain brings energy and love to all they undertake. These are the people who, having once given their word, will fulfill their commitment, even though it be to their own disadvantage. The desire to serve of Centaury, the determination of Oak, the enthusiasm of Verain, together they would make a powerful trinity.

While history may write glowing reports of the deeds of its most famous Vervain sons, in everyday circumstances they can be difficult to live with! Like a terrier who will not let go, they worry and fret and run round in circles, refusing to rest until they feel that they have accomplished something. Frustrations can lead to sleeplessness — at times the thoughts going round and round in their head can make them difficult to distinguish from White Chestnut. White Chestnut thoughts are random, related to everyday affairs of no real importance, except maybe to them. Verain thoughts are directed towards things which need to be accomplished. Impatiens and Vervain are also similar in that both remedies tend to be quick in thought and action. Impatiens prefers to work alone, Vervain in company.

Chancellor gave another quotation from Dr. Bach, which is of importance: "They have the enthusiasm and excitement of the possession of great knowledge". Scientists and inventors may be just as excited about discoveries relating to the physical universe as a devotee with spiritual revelation. We understand why this remedy finds its place in the last group. These people are not merely treading the old familiar way; they are beginning to break new ground — or, at least, they believe they are. The inspiration of discovery brings with it great enthusiasm.

While sharing this insight and enthusiasm with others is a worthy aim, we must respect other people's individuality as much as we ask, and expect, them to respect ours. In the same way that we do not appreciate other people preaching to, or trying to convert, us, we must not try to impose our way on others. It is a hard lesson to learn when we are convinced that what we have to offer is to the other's benefit, even necessary to save the world, or, at least, the environment.

Vervain holds a precarious place between two very dominating remedies, Chicory and Vine. Vervain cannot impose their views in the same way as Chicory, because one cannot manipulate people outside the home as easily as one's relatives. Nevertheless, they can exercise emotional blackmail with every bit as much finesse as Chicory. Instead of saying, "You will upset me very much if you do not do as I wish," they say, "You will upset God very much if you do not do as I wish". They may not express it in quite such a forthright way (although they might), nevertheless the rightness they are claiming for their position is not merely the rightness of whether it is time to trade in the family car or cold enough to wear a sweater, it is the rightness of ideas, a speaking on behalf of the Almighty, as though they were in some way privy to His thoughts, more so than other human beings.

Through meditation, insight, revelation or plain good living, no doubt some people are more "in tune" than others. Over the centuries, Vervain people have been an inspiration and the world owes them much. But we must not forget that every privilege brings with it its associated responsibility.

We look back to Vervain's partner and find it to be Aspen. We may remember how the soul in its Aspen state was so fearful, especially of 'other-worldly' things. Now, instead of shivering in its shoes at every breath of wind, Vervain faces the world, and the world beyond, fearlessly. Let the wind blow, let the storm rage. Vervain will stand firm.

Great progress has been made. Proceed with caution.

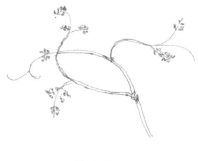

Vine
(Vitis vinifera)

As Chicory and Vervain before them, Vine people are very sure of their own opinion. They also think it could be "of benefit if others thought and acted in the same way, as they direct". In other words, Vine are dictators, whether in their own home or on the world stage.

Ask any group of people to name a dictator and the answer will instantly come — "Hitler". I have never yet had a class name Hitler as an example of Vervain, yet, in his early days, Hitler was Vervain. He swept the people of Germany along with him on a tide of enthusiasm, such as has never been seen anywhere else in the world. He exhorted them to share his vision. It may be hard for us today to understand how such an unprepossessing man could exert such an influence; that he did, despite his rather ordinary looks, speaks volumes for his magnetic personality. We all know the end of the story.

Unfortunately, in life, Vine often does follow Vervain.

Some people are born Vine, others become Vine when their enthusiasm for their cause deafens them to any argument. It must be realized that it is impossible to become Vine alone. In a corporate or national situation, Vine needs an army of supporters (either literally or figuratively). Even within the home, Vine can only dominate those who allow themselves to be dominated.

There are big Vines and little Vines, but wherever they are found they have one thing in common. They climb over others, having a stranglehold over those very people upon whom they depend for support and for their own development and fruitfulness.

Hitler may be the best known example of the transition from Vervain to Vine, but there are many others. The post-war years saw several examples of self-proclaimed religious leaders who gathered around them a band of enthusiastic followers, over whom they exerted so great a degree of domination that these followers chose death rather than desertion (Jonestown, 1978, Waco, Texas, 1993).

Death rather than desertion — we need people who can inspire this degree of loyalty to defend us in times of war. As Dr. Bach said, "They may be of great value in emergency". If the ship is sinking, pray there is a Vine on board! They give orders so naturally, so confidently, so authoritatively, that people will automatically obey them and many lives may be saved.

Within a home or office situation, a true Vine person may be able to impose their will on their unfortunate underlings by sheer unpleasantness and bad temper, but within a larger social environment this would rarely be tolerated by sufficient people to enable the Vine person to establish their authority. They are forced to suppress or disguise their dominating beneath a veneer of amiability. Many show one side at work, the other at home.

Leaders are essential, not only in human society, but also in the animal kingdom. Vine personalities are necessary but to exert authority without abusing power is no easy task. Many may unwittingly progress from Vervain to Vine over a number of years as the admiration they inspire in others, coupled with their undoubted capabilities, wreaks its subtle damage.

A Vine person is unlikely to be insulted if you tell them of your diagnosis because they see nothing wrong in being sure of their own abilities, of being a leader among men. Rather, they feel complimented. It is quite possible that many Vine people will be unaware of their state, believing themselves to be Verain. Others know, and are proud. They want to lead. They perceive their authoritative nature as a gift — and perhaps it is!

Both Vervain and Vine are happiest working as part of a team. Neither relishes being alone. The difference is that Verain leads from the front, by example, taking on greater burden of work than any other member of the team. Vine leads from above. They direct the work of others, allocating tasks so that their own workload is kept to a manageable level. The true Vine person rarely suffers nervous exhaustion because of this ability to delegate.

I spoke of Chicory being the remedy of the matriarch. Vine is the remedy of the patriarch. Of course, such gender stereotyping is not absolute, but it serves to illustrate a point. Chicory people rarely resort to violence. They obtain their objective by emotional manipulation. The duty they claim is a duty of care — from those for whom they themselves are caring or have cared. The duty claimed by the Vine person is that of obedience. They recognize their position as one of authority, be they parent or employer, sergeant or sovereign, which means, ipso facto, that the other person's position is rightfully one of obedience. The

Vine person will resort to violence, if necessary, in the belief that the end justifies the means.

As Chicory was the vehicle for bringing to perfection the divine aspect of love, so Vine is the vehicle for perfecting the divine aspect of will.

One image of the Heavenly Father is of that Being in whom reposes all power, but who refrains from force or compulsion, allowing his children to develop their own abilities and nature. How hard it is to have authority and power, but to use these not for the self, but only for the benefit of those over whom one rules.

The ability to lead, to take responsibility, this must be achieved by all human beings during the course of their evolution, be it in small or great matters. The task is to know when to direct, when to encourage andwhen to leave well alone. Perfect Wisdom is the only guide.

Vine offers a total contrast to its partner, Cherry Plum. While Cherry Plum was in a state of panic, fearing loss of control over the current situation, whatever that may be, Vine is the complete opposite. Vine has more control over their situation and surroundings than any other remedy.

You may remember that I said there were no more suicidal remedies after Elm and you may ask, "What about Hitler? He killed himself." The Vine person will not commit suicide while in the Vine state, while they have control over their life and the situation in which they are placed. If they lose control over their empire, the Vine person may revert, temporarily, to a Cherry Plum state. Their mind is overstrained, their reason gives way, they commit the fearful and dreaded act, not wished for and known to be wrong. The Vine personality, in a Cherry Plum state, is probably the highest suicide risk of all.

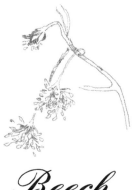

Beech
(Fagus sylvatica)

We come now to the penultimate remedy. The soul is nearing the completion of its journey.

Beech is the remedy of final adjustments, of dotting the i's and crossing the t's. The Beech person is acutely aware of every imperfection in the world around them, from the picture which hangs slightly crookedly on the wall to the state of the hole in the ozone layer.

This is the remedy which strives to understand, and work with, the laws of the Universe. It realizes the perfection of creation, the perfect balance in, and of, all things. The slightest deviation from this balance and perfection offends the sensitive soul.

If the perfectionism of Beech was directed solely towards themselves, there might be no problem. However, Beech strives to reach perfection in all things which causes them to be critical of other people and things which they perceive as being less than perfect.

Dr. Bach tells us that these people need to be more tolerant and understanding of the different way in which each individual and all things are working towards their own final perfection.

I find these last few words very significant. It seems more than a co-incidence that Dr. Bach should use the phrase "final perfection" in relation to this remedy, and this remedy alone, so close to the end of the journey. I feel it to be one more clue to the master plan in his presentation of the remedies to us. He urged us to understand that, although much appears to be wrong, there is good growing within all things.

In our Mimulus state, we feared worldly things, felt ourselves threatened by them. Having reached the Beech state, we have overcome this fear. We no longer feel personally threatened, but the Beech person is still over-concerned with daily living, with worldly problems and defects in relation to themselves, the world, the Universe and its Creator.

As with all the remedies, the Beech state can manifest on many different levels, from the most petty to the most profound. We experience each state in the manner appropriate to our level of development. Continual opportunity is offered us through multitudinous experiences to perfect our performance until eventually the perfect act and actor become One and the soul achieves its ultimate goal.

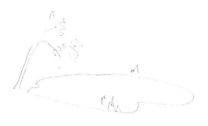

Rock Water

And so we reach our final remedy, doubly interesting because it is the only one not drawn from the plant kingdom, although present in all. Water has long been associated with purification and Dr. Bach found in the waters of a spring with healing properties the remedy to bring his work to completion.

Rock Water is the remedy for the soul which is practicing self-discipline. It has left behind the desire to control, organize and perfect others; its efforts are now concentrated solely towards the self.

In the less evolved Rock Water person, this effort may still involve some selfishness. The Rock Water people will subject themselves to whatever hardships they consider necessary to attain their life's goal. Striving for excellence day after day, week after week, year after year of unremitting effort is not considered too big a price for that one moment of glory when they achieve their ultimate aim. They do desire to be better than others and will not allow others to stand in their way, demanding support and understanding from any who would wish to be counted among their select circle of friends.

And yet these people are not selfish in that the base of their desire to reach the pinnacle lies in a desire to overcome adversity, not an opponent. Whether it be the rocky face of Mount Everest, or the determined face of a sporting opponent which confronts them, it is their own physical and mental limitations which they are striving to conquer. In the evolved soul, this remedy reflects the letting go of the desire to impose one's will on others, that most divine of all sacrifices, for even God does not impose his/her will on any of his/her creatures.

The spiritual seeker willingly renounces any earthly joys which stand in the way of the greatest of all joys — Self/God Realization. They do not try to impose their discipline on others, although they will teach and encourage others, if asked. "They hope to be examples which will appeal to others who may then follow their ideas and be better as a result." What greater good can there be in life than this? The saint, the guru, the Avatar: blessed Rock Water, each and every one. From the terror of Rock Rose, we travel the path to total self-mastery with Rock Water, attaining the final divine gift of Wisdom.

The disciple, having accepted discipline, passes on to a far greater Discipleship than is granted to us here below.

And so we come to the end of our
Journeyings

May the blessings of the seven beautiful gifts
of healing be yours

Bibliography

Bach, E. (1931) The Twelve Healers. London. The C. W. Daniel Co. Ltd.

Bach, E. (1933) The Twelve Healers and Other Remedies. London. The C. W. Daniel Co. Ltd.

Bernard J. (ed.) Collected Writings of Edward Bach. Hereford. Flower Remedy Programme.

Chancellor, P. (1971) Handbook of the Bach Flower Remedies. Saffron Walden. The C. W. Daniel Co. Ltd.

Clarke, J.. H. (1990) The Therapeutics of Cancer. (Indian edition) New Delhi. B. Jain Publishers Ltd.

Close, S. (1982) The Genius of Homoeopathy. (Indian edition) New Dehli. B. Jain Publishers Ltd.

Cooper, R. (1990) Cancer and Cancer Treatment. (Indian edition) New Delhi. B. Jain Publishers Ltd.

Frankl, V. (1959) Man's Search for Meaning. New York. Washington Square Press.

Howard, J. and Ramsall, J. (1990) The Original Writings of Edward Bach. Saffron Walden. The C. W. Daniel Co. Ltd.

Milne, A. A. (1972) Disobedience: When we were very young. London. Mehuen Children's Books.

Weeks, N. (1940) The Medical Discoveries of Edward Bach, Physician. Saffron Walden, England. The C. W. Daniel Co. Ltd.

Godde's

Paperchase

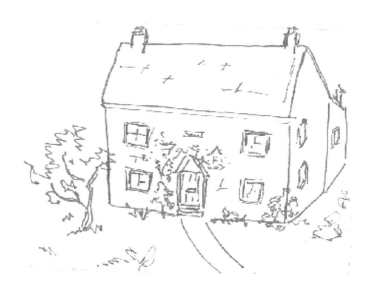

An allegorical tale dedicated to Dr. Bach and his wonderful Flowers

Chapter One

In which Queen Chicory has a headache and Wizard Elm has a busy night

Once upon a time, long, long ago, in a land far, far away, there lived a king. Now, this king was a good king. Indeed, he was a very good king. Nothing delighted the king more than the thought that all his subjects should be as happy as he. Nothing distressed him more than the thought that not all his subjects could be as rich as he, for, although he was a good king, he was not a stupid king and he knew as well as anyone that one of the duties of a king was to be rich.

A king must live in a castle, wear fine clothes and have a crown of gold upon his head. All of these things, King Vervain did, for, as I have already told you, he was a good king, but he did wish at times that the crown of gold was not quite so heavy, or so cold to wear in the winter. It did tend to give him a headache, but this he gladly suffered, or, at least, he grumbled about but rarely, because he knew that to wear a crown was the right thing to do.

When he awoke in the morning, the first thought that

entered King Vervain's mind was "What can I do to-day to make my people happy?" and the last thought he had before he fell asleep at night was, "What can I do to-morrow to make my people happier still?"

Each time King Vervain met one of his subjects, he greeted them with a smile and a merry "Hi!" and they greeted him with a merry, "Hi!" in return. This happy custom had lead to his kingdom being known as the Kingdom of Merry Hi Hi!

Now, I wish I could tell you that all the people in the kingdom of Merry Hi Hi were as happy as the king. Indeed, most of them were happy, as least when things were going well, but there was one person in the kingdom who was hardly ever happy, even when things were going very well indeed. That person was Duke Vine. Duke Vine wanted to be king so that he could tell everybody what to do and punish them if they did not do as they were told. He thought King Vervain was very silly to want to make everyone else happy. "What is the point," thought Duke Vine to himself, "in being the most powerful person in the kingdom if you do not use your power to make sure that everybody else does exactly what you want them to do?"

Of course, Duke Vine was a duke and dukes are Very Important People. They live in castles, too, although their castles are not as big as the king's castle. They are rich, and have lots and lots of servants, but they do not wear a golden crown on their head. And, of course, most importantly of all, they have to do what the king tells them to do,

Being the second most important person in the kingdom, Duke Vine could boss just about everybody else about, and this he did every day. He kept his poor servants scurrying here and scurrying there, doing his bidding on every little thing, but still he was not happy.

If the servants were too slow, or made a mistake, he would punish them severely, by making them sweep the floor they had already swept ten times more, or run round and round the castle wall, which was his very favourite punishment because it ensured that his servants were the fittest servants in the whole land! But still he was not happy.

King Vervain sighed when he saw how unhappy Duke Vine was and tried to make him feel better by giving him more servants to wait on him, but somehow this never made Duke Vine smile for very long.

Poor King Vervain! He tried to make Duke Vine happy because his own beautiful wife, Queen Chicory, was Duke Vine's sister! Now, if Duke Vine was bossy, Queen Chicory was bossier still! But she was very clever because she often made it look as though she were the one who was helping, while all the time it was she who was getting her own way.

Only last week, she held a christening party for the baby son of one of the knights at the castle. Everyone said how generous she was, although, of course, it was her servants who did all the work and her husband, the king, who paid the bill. In truth, she wanted to be godmother to the child, but did not want the bother of travelling to the knight's castle, which she considered small and dark compared with the palace, which, of course, it was. So everybody else had travelled to her castle and Queen Chicory basked in the sunshine of everyone's thanks for her generosity!

King Vervain did everything he could to make his Queen happy, but, like her brother, Queen Chicory could always find something not to her liking. Sometimes King Vervain would think to himself that if there was one thing which could spoil his happiness when he sat down to a banquet in the Great Hall, it was the fact that he had to be seated between his wife, Queen Chicory, and his brother-in-law, Duke Vine!

It would have been a great treat for him if he could, just once, have sat at a table with the young knights, or even the servants, and join in their happy laughter, but King Vervain knew that as a good king he must sit at the head of the table with the two other most important people on either side of him, so he shifted his crown a little and settled down to enjoy the evening. Soon the Court Jester, Agrimony, would arrive; his witty jokes and humorous ballads would ensure an evening full of laughter and song.

King Vervain was not the type of person to allow anything to spoil his enthusiasm for life for long. As he sank his teeth into the juicy meat and drank the sweet wine, he smiled and looked around the Great Hall, pleased to see everyone enjoying their meal. He was thankful that the people of his kingdom were at peace and as happy as those of any kingdom in the world.

King Vervain always felt better when he went to speak to Wizard Elm. He enjoyed going to the underground cellars where Wizard Elm studied his spells and made his magic potions. It was the only place in the entire kingdom where King Vervain felt he did not have to carry all the responsibility. He could tell his problems to someone else and it was up to Wizard Elm to find the answer.

Wizard Elm's heart sank when he heard King Vervain approach. "Oh dear!" he said to himself. "Queen Chicory must be feeling ill again. I have tried every spell and potion in my book and still the Queen does not recover. I believe she enjoys being ill. Even Duke Vine fusses over her, which is more than he does over anyone else. She has everyone dancing attendance on her, with all her complaints."

Wizard Elm was wise, as all wizards are. He knew that sometimes being fussed over and cared for was more important that being well, so he patiently promised to do his best to have a very special brew ready for Queen Chicory to take first thing in the morning.

Another long night! Besides the medicine for the Queen, he must prepare a soothing drink for Master Larch, who had a nasty cold, and another for Chestnut Bud, the gnome, whose cough was no better, although Wizard Elm did feel that this was his own fault for spending quite so much time down by the lake talking to the nymph, Water Violet.

If he had told Chestnut Bud once, he had told him a hundred times, gnomes are no good at swimming. Now, besides the cough, Chestnut Bud was complaining of aches in his joints. Would he never learn!

Sometimes Wizard Elm felt that the responsibility of keeping everyone in the kingdom in good health was really too much! But if he didn't, who would?

Wizard Elm lit another candle and turned over the page of his book.

Chapter Two

In which Princess Clematis takes a tumble and Sir Scleranthus has to make a descision

While King Verain, Queen Chicory, Duke Vine and all the other people of the kingdom of Merry Hi Hi (except Wizard Elm, who was still working on Queen Chicory's potion) snuggled down in their warm beds for a peaceful night's sleep, high in a cave on the mountain top, dragon Red Chestnut was watching over the sleeping mortals.

It was the time of day (or, rather, night) that Red Chestnut liked the best. As the sun went down he watched the windows of the cottages light up with the flickering of candles and fires in their hearths. While the mortals were busy cooking and eating their evening meal, telling each other tales of their day and preparing for bed, all was quiet in the streets and fields below. Red Chestnut was able to watch the smoke rising from the chimneys, making patterns as it twisted and circled with each passing breeze.

Like all dragons, Red Chestnut could breathe out fire and smoke and he liked to play at making the same pattern with his smoke as the playful breezes made with the smoke rising from the chimneys below. This was not as easy as it might sound, particularly as the patterns were never the same twice, but with hours of practice, Red Chestnut was becoming quite skilled and was very proud of his achievements.

He looked across at his friend, the unicorn, already fast asleep. "Not surprising. White Chestnut is never still for a minute during the day. Not that he will sleep all night. After a short rest, he will be awake again, leaping from point to point as he plays over the rocky mountainside. Up to mischief, as usual, no doubt."

Red Chestnut was troubled. Like King Vervain, his dearest wish was for everyone to be safe and happy, but, like Queen Chicory, he was in a constant state of anxiety about all sorts of things lest something should go wrong.

While Queen Chicory only worried about problems which were happening at the time, Red Chestnut worried about all sorts of things that might happen, but usually didn't, which was fortunate, because if all the things Red Chestnut worried about did actually happen, King Vervain's kingdom would be a sorry place indeed!

Now, it must be understood that Red Chestnut had good cause to be so anxious. What I have not yet explained to you is that Red Chestnut did not live in the cave at the mountain top all alone. Not only did he share the cave with White Chestnut, the mischievous unicorn, he also lived there with three very bad fairies!

Of course, they did not consider that they were bad. On the contrary, they were of the opinion that all the bad deeds they did brought interest and excitement into the lives of the people of Merry Hi Hi, "for," they said to themselves, "if nothing exciting or interesting ever happened, how boring life would be!"

While he was lazily watching the smoke rising from the chimneys of the cottages below, Red Chestnut was listening to Rock Rose telling Cherry Plum how that day she had caused a rock to fall from the edge of the cliff just as Princess Clematis was walking by. This had caused Princess Clematis to tumble down the cliff, where she lay trapped on a narrow ledge for two whole hours before her cries were heard by the young knight, Sir Scleranthus, who happened to be riding by.

Sir Scleranthus could not make up his mind whether to climb down the cliff himself to rescue the Princess, or to go for help, wasting valuable time trying to make up his mind which was the best course to follow, while Princess Clematis was lying on the ledge, absolutely terrified lest it, too, should give way and she should fall to the valley below.

Rock Rose was delighted with the result of her scheme and told Cherry Plum that this would be an experience Princess Clematis would remember for the rest of her life, which was some achievement since Princess Clematis was generally very forgetful.

Eventually, Sir Scleranthus had ridden back on his faithful horse, Centaury, to fetch Mr. Oak, the blacksmith, who was the strongest man in the kingdom. It did not take Blacksmith Oak long to rescue Princess Clematis from the ledge, although he did give her a sound scolding for not watching where she was going.

If only Princess Clematis would concentrate on what she was doing, instead of living in a world of dreams, she would not have so many mishaps. To the practical blacksmith, dreaming was for night time. Building castles in the air when you should be learning your lessons or watching your step was a foolishness which could only lead to trouble.

Princess Clematis thanked Mr. Oak most sincerely for rescuing her and promised that she would try to be better in the future, but it was hard to concentrate when so many ideas were constantly filling her mind.

"I had been wondering about what o'clock it was" explained the contrite Princess, "when it occurred to me that it should be possible to make a sun dial small enough to tie to one's wrist so that one could tell the time of day wherever one went."

"What folly," chided the practical Mr. Oak "a time piece so small that you could carry it around with you! Foolish, foolish child! What will you think of next?"

Now the bad fairy, Rock Rose, was planning what trouble she could cause. Her younger sister, Cherry Plum, and her daughter Mimulus were eagerly joining in the conversation. Like Rock Rose, Cherry Plum wanted to take her time to create some really big trouble, but the youngster was less fussy. She amused herself, not by creating big troubles for humans, but by stirring up lots of little ones.

Mimulus was especially fond of upsetting the children of the village. She delighted in making them afraid of all sorts of things, such as going to bed in the dark, of forgetting their lessons at school and of taking the medicine which Wizard Elm prepared for them when they were sick. It was so easy to make the children afraid of things which were really good for them!

On Fridays, when the school teacher, Mr. Gentian, tested their work, Mimulus made the children so afraid that they quite forgot all the things they had learned! Mr. Gentian could never understand why, after all his careful teaching on

Monday, Tuesday, Wednesday and Thursday, the children seemed to remember so little on Friday. It really was very disheartening!

At times he felt like giving up trying to teach the children altogether, but then something would happen which showed him that there were times when they did learn, and he would cheer up again. "After all," he would say to himself, "a tree does not grow in a day. From little acorns, mighty oak trees grow."

Thinking of oak trees reminded him that he really would have to be more strict with Mr. Oak's daughter, Wild Rose. She was such a lazy child, would not do anything if she could avoid it. Mind you, Mr. Gentian did feel very sorry for Wild Rose. She used to be a happy child before her mother died.

Now she seemed to have lost interest in everything. Her father, steady and reliable, worked long hours in the village forge. He had little time to spend with Wild Rose. Even Queen Chicory felt sorry for her and had arranged for her eldest daughter, Princess Holly, to befriend her.

It was a strange friendship. At first, Princess Holly had been angry at being told to make friends with the blacksmith's daughter, but in reality they had much in common. Both were angry because of something in their lives over which they had no control. Wild Rose was angry because her mother had died. Princess Holly was angry because, as a girl, she would not rule the kingdom after her father died. That honour would go to her younger brother, Prince Walnut, of whom she was fiercely jealous. And so these two young people, the one so energetic and the other so lazy, found comfort in each other's company.

Chapter Three

In which Prince Walnut looks forward and Mr. Honeysuckle looks back

Beneath the castle roof that night, Sir Scleranthus also tossed and turned in his bed and awoke to greet the light of day with a heavy heart. He felt he had been a failure the day before because he had not rescued the little Princess Clematis single handed. What was the good of being a knight in shining armour if you could not rescue a damsel in distress?

Now, I need to explain to you that Sir Scleranthis was indeed a knight in shining armour. Very shining — because his armour was very new! Only a short time ago, he had performed all the needs of valour necessary to satisfy the requirements for being made a knight. Scleranthus had shown his skills in horsemanship and jousting before the King and all the Knights of the Realm. It had been the proudest moment of his life when he had knelt before King Vervain who had touched him on either shoulder with his great sword and said, "Rise, Sir Scleranthus". Now he had his own Coat of Arms and would lead soldiers into battle in the event that King Vervain ever declared war on one of the neighbouring kingdoms, which Sir Scleranthus had to admit to himself, somewhat ruefully, was highly unlikely!

Nevertheless, in preparation for this event, however unlikely, the blacksmith, Mr. Oak, had forged a suit of shining armour, made especially for him, which was the pride of his life. Every week he oiled and polished its gleaming plates of steel, unable to make up his mind whether he wanted his suit to remain in its pristine state or whether he would be more proud of it in years to come when it bore the marks of many blows gathered upon the field of battle — or at least in the jousting ring!

"What," he asked himself, "is the use of being good at jousting if one cannot climb down a rock face to rescue a terrified princess?" That he had been instrumental in bringing about her rescue did little to repair his dented pride. To make matters worse, it was only last week that King Verain had summoned him to the castle to take over the instruction of his son, Prince Walnut, who was now old enough to be trained for knighthood and needed to learn all the skills of which Sir Scleranthis had so short a time ago shown himself to be so proficient.

Thinking of King Verain reminded Sir Scleranthus that he was to ride with the King this morning before breakfast. King Verain always woke early and enjoyed an hour or two's ride over the fields and through the forests before returning to the castle for a hearty breakfast and whatever made King Vervain feel good, he was sure would make everyone else feel good too, so he always invited his knights to join him for his early morning ride. He would have liked to invite the villagers too, but they were already busy working in the fields.

Sir Scleranthus hurried down to the stables where he found Prince Walnut already mounted on his horse. Sir Scleranthus took the reins of his stallion from the groom and gracefully leapt into the saddle. Within minutes, they were across the drawbridge and galloping freely over the meadow. As he breathed in the crisp morning air and felt the first rays of the sun warm his skin, he could not help reflecting that perhaps King Vervain was right after all. Reluctant as one might be to follow his advice, one usually did benefit in the end. Indeed, it was difficult for anybody to feel downcast for long in the presence of his good-natured enthusiasm.

Prince Walnut was not so sure. "It's all very well for you, Scleranthus," he said. "You will only live at the castle for a short time. When you marry, you will have a home of your own. But as for me, I am a prince. I cannot escape. My life is planned for me, almost every minute of the day. And for years into the future! I cannot even choose my own bride, but must marry the princess my father chooses for me. How I wish I could break free from all the constraints which surround me and be like one of the villagers."

"And how the villagers wish they could be like you," laughed Sir Scleranthus, "with all your fine clothes, good food to eat every day and servants to do your bidding."

"'Tis true," agreed Prince Walnut. "How rarely are we satisfied with our lot in life. When I was young, I was happy because I was spoilt and had no worries. But now, I must learn to read, and to write, to ride a horse while wearing heavy armour, to joust and fight like a grown man, and yet I am scarcely more than a boy and have not my father's sturdy frame."

"No," agreed Sir Sclearnthus, "you are more finely built like your mother, Queen Chicory. But cheer up! This stage of your life will soon pass. Once you are fully grown into a man, you will no longer have to prove that you are one! If you prefer to watch the tournaments rather than participate in them, no one will care. It is just a stage of your life through which you must pass."

"You are right, I know," replied Prince Walnut. "It's just that some stages in life are harder to endure than others."

"Race you back to the castle," cried Scleranthus. He felt his horse, Centaury, respond to his call. "What beautiful creatures horses are," he thought to himself, "so big, so strong and so graceful. Yet how rarely they want their own way. They are ever ready to do the slightest bidding of their master, be it depth of winter or height of summer; they walk, gallop, turn this way or that, their joy being in doing what is asked of them, without thought of their own desires. There is no other creature so willing or obedient. No, not even you, my faithful hound", he said, as his dog, Way-to-go, came out to greet him.

He patted the horse and dog in turn, unable to decide which one was more in need of his attention. He remembered well his seventh birthday, when his father had given him the hound as a present.

"You are old enough now, my son, to venture alone outside the confines of our grounds. Should you ever lose your way when out in the countryside, do not be alarmed. The dog will know the way to go."

And so he had called him Way-to-go and, true to his name, Way-to-go had never let him down. When he hesitated at a fork in the road, not knowing which path to follow, faithful Way-to-go would know the way and bring him safely back home.

Young Larch, the groom, was waiting at the stables to rub

Centaury down after the early morning ride. Larch was the son of Mr. and Mrs. Gorse from the farm down by the lake. His grandfather, Mr. Honeysuckle, now old and retired from farming, kept the village Inn.

"Prince Walnut," cried Sir Scleranthus, "after breakfast let us go to the Sythe and Sickle and pass the hour of day with old Mr. Honeysuckle. He has such tales to tell of days gone by. I love to listen to them."

"Indeed, so do I," replied Prince Walnut, "except when I am waiting to be served with some hot mead on a cold winter's day. Even being a prince does not enable me to escape from some of old Mr. Honeysuckle's stories! I do declare that he might be Old Father Time himself, for the past is more real to him than the present. It is fortunate for him that nobody in the kingdom can make mead as he can, else he would have no customers!"

As expected, they found Mr. Honeysuckle sitting on a bench outside his cottage, with a jug of mead in his hand.

"Good day to you, young gentlemen," he greeted them. "And how did you enjoy your ride this morning? I saw you galloping across the meadows. In my young day, I would have led the lot of you. I had this beautiful horse, as black as the night he was; he could out-race any horse in the land."

Walnut and Scleranthus let the old man ramble on, happy in his memories, while they enjoyed the warmth of the sunshine and the sweet smell of the honeysuckle, which, like its namesake, rambled all over the place. It came as quite a surprise when, some time later, Sir Scleranthus realized that Mr. Honeysuckle had returned to the present and was talking about his grandson, Larch.

"So kind of you to take Larch into your service, Sir," he was saying. "He does so much admire you, but I keep telling him, 'admiration is not much use without imitation.' I wish he would put more effort into being like you instead of talking about you. He lacks confidence in his own abilities. I tell him that in order to triumph, it's not enough just to try, you need some umph as well. Mind you, I blame that father of his. Never could understand why my daughter married that grumpy fellow. Always down in the dumps is our Mr. Gorse. Can't be good for young Larch to be living with someone who is always so depressed. Mind you, he has had more than his share of troubles in life but he should not let them get him down so. Other people get over life's set backs, so why can't Mr. Gorse?"

Prince Walnut and Sir Scleranthus settled back to listen to the old man recount yet again, all the many and various troubles which had befallen the Gorse family As always, he blamed the wicked fairies of the mountains for causing all the problems.

"Do you believe in the fairies?" asked Sir Sclelranthus.

"Wizard Elm does and that is good enough for me," the old man replied. "There are many spirits and creatures in the mountain which we hardly ever see."

"Once when I was young, I did think I saw the unicorn," agreed Sir Scleranthus, "but I never see it now."

"Ah, that is because you sold your baby teeth to the Tooth Fairy," replied Mr. Honeysuckle. "I remember my grandfather telling me that the little ones can see the fairy folk, but once they sell their teeth to the Tooth Fairy, they lose their innocence and can no longer see the spirits. I don't know if it is true, but that is what he did say."

Before returning to the castle, Prince Walnut took one last look at the beautiful mountain which soared above the valley, its top hidden by the wisps of cloud (or was that smoke from the dragon's cave?). Its slopes were covered by graceful trees between which he could catch glimpses of the river as it tumbled over the rocks, in places cascading down the mountain side in the most beautiful of water falls. As the river wended its way down the mountain, it became broader and deeper and its waters more gentle. How peaceful the lake looked now, nestled at the base of the mountain, with the sky and the mountain peaks reflected in its deep calm waters.

Prince Walnut wished he could spend all day sitting outside the Sythe and Sickle listening to old Mr. Honeysuckle's stories, but he knew it was time to return. Mr. Gentian would have finished giving the village children their morning lessons and would be waiting for him in the castle school room!

Chapter Four

In which a gnome is captivated by a nymph and fails to learn a lesson

Meanwhile, down at the lake, things were not as peaceful as they seemed. Beneath the surface the fish were ceaselessly swimming, darting to and fro in their endless search for food — while at the same time endeavouring not to become some other creature's next meal!

In the centre of the lake, aloof from all the activity below, the beautiful nymph, Water Violet, sat quietly dangling her pretty toes in the water. She loved to watch the birds as they swooped over the lake, the bees as they buzzed around the blossoms, the butterflies flitting from flower to flower and the frogs as they jumped from lily pad to lily pad. She, alone, seemed unmoved among all the hustle and bustle and her quiet serenity fascinated the gnome, Chestnut Bud.

As you know, gnomes are hardworking, friendly people, always ready for a good yarn over a tankard of ale and a good beefsteak pie of an evening. Working, talking, eating and sleeping, those are the things gnomes do best. One of the things gnomes do not do very well, as I mentioned before, is swim! None of the other gnomes, who lived in the banks beside the lake, had any interest in swimming at all, but then, none of the other gnomes were married to Chestnut Bud's wife, Heather!

Now, Chestnut Bud was very fond of his wife. She was a good woman, definitely the best cook in the whole of Merry Hi Hi, but she never stopped talking! No incident in Mistress Heather's day was too trivial for her to recount at great length to any other gnome, if she could induce them to engage in conversation with her. Mistress Heather only had one topic of conversation — herself! Maybe this was a good thing, because so long as she was talking about herself, she wasn't talking about other people!

Be that as it may, Chestnut Bud was glad to escape at times to share the quietness of Water Violet's company. No one ever knew if Water Violet was as glad to see Chestnut Bud as he was to see her, for she never said. In fact, she said very little at all, but there was no one else as good as she at listening, so many people sought her company. No wonder she spent most of her time on a leaf in the middle of the lake!

Chestnut Bud could see his wife talking to one of the other gnomes, no doubt swapping recipes for tonight's dinner. Ah! Whatever other faults Mistress Heather might have, no one could say she was not the best cook in the district. Even the King's own cook had been known to ask her advice on special dishes for banquets at the castle! Already the smell of beefsteak pie was wafting over the water, but what would be for dessert? Apple dumplings and cream? Treacle pudding? Chocolate fudge cake with caramel sauce?

Chestnut Bud heaved a sigh of contented anticipation — which was a mistake because, with a loud pop, yet another button flew off his waistcoat! Oh dear! He knew he was getting too fat and kept promising himself to cut down on his meals, but, somehow, when confronted with one of Mistress Heather's dinners, all he had learned from previous experience seemed to leave him, and he tucked in heartily. He would start his diet tomorrow, really he would!

Chestnut Bud pondered which would be worse — going without Mistress Heather's wonderful food so that he could fit into his clothes again, or going to visit Mr. Mustard, the tailor, to be measured for a new suit? He wondered what mood Mr. Mustard would be in just now. Some days he seemed quite chirpy but at other times it was as though a black cloud had descended on him. He had a face like a thundercloud and a temper to match!

At times these bad moods would last for days or weeks on end. The trouble was that no one ever knew what type of mood he would be in, because there never seemed to be any reason for them. Wizard Elm told him to eat plenty of mustard as that would be good for him. Chestnut Bud was never sure whether that was how he got his name, or whether it was just a co-incidence. He never dared to ask and it probably didn't matter anyway, because, mustard or no mustard, Mr. Mustard's moods seemed to be getting worse with every passing year.

Chestnut Bud decided he would worry about his clothes tomorrow. The problem now was whether or not he should risk swimming out to join Water Violet. Wizard Elm had spoken to him very sternly about the foolishness of his behaviour when he brought the cough syrup and the ointment for his aching knees.

Chestnut Bud felt sure that the cough syrup was quite the nastiest Wizard Elm had ever prepared for him — trying to teach him a lesson no doubt — but he swallowed it all the same and rubbed the ointment very thoroughly all over his knees before he went to bed. The fumes made his eyes water so much that he wondered if he had caught Larch's cold.

His wife complained, too. In fact, she had declared that she could not sleep in the room while it smelt so strongly of the ointment and had gone next door to her sister's house for the night, which might be why Chestnut Bud was feeling so well this morning.

Out of the corner of his eye, Chestnut Bud saw that Mistress Heather had finished talking to her neighbour and was heading in his direction. Without thinking any further, he slipped into the clear water of the lake.

The sun might be shining, but the waters of the lake, which came from the mountain stream, were very cold. Chestnut Bud caught his breath as he coughed and spluttered his way ungracefully towards the pad on which Water Violet was sitting.

Water Violet smiled to herself as she saw him coming and watched while he struggled to heave himself up onto the slippery leaf. Not for the first time, Chestnut Bud wished gnomes had wings!

Once settled, he chatted happily to Water Violet, who was quite a good conversationalist once she got started. She had an immense store of tales which she had been told by the many people who sought her company over the years and her keen interest in anything unusual or out of the ordinary ensured that she could always captivate her audience, when she chose to do so.

One of the tales she told that afternoon was so funny, and Chestnut Bud laughed so heartily, he fell off the leaf and drenched his clothes, which had nearly dried in the sun. The sun was losing its warmth and Chestnut Bud knew it was time for him to paddle his way through the now VERY cold waters of the lake, back to Yummy Yummy Cottage, from where the smell of tonight's dinner was calling him home. Beefsteak pie and ? Yes, definitely. Chocolate fudge pudding with caramel sauce. His favourite! What a good thing he had decided not to start his diet until tomorrow!

Chapter Five

In which White Chestnut causes a mischief and Princess Clematis has another idea

Gnome Chestnut Bud was not the only person who smelt Mistress Heather's dinner cooking that night. Out for an evening stroll on the battlements of the castle, King Vervain had also smelt the delicious aroma and it had reminded him that it was time to start preparing for his son's birthday party. Prince Walnut would be twelve come this Hallow E'en. Why King Vervain should feel so proud that his son had been born at this time, when he had nothing to do with it, it was hard to explain, but he did.

What father would not be proud to have a son born at Hallow E'en and a daughter born on Christmas Day! With her dark, fiery eyes and her sharp tongue, she was well named Princess Holly, for there were few in the Palace who had not been on the receiving end of her prickly tongue when she was angry — which was more often than King Vervain would have liked.

Princess Clematis had been born just two and a half years after Prince Walnut, on May Day. At times it did trouble King Vervain a little that all three of the children had such special birthdays. He suspected that the herbal brew which Wizard Elm had concocted for Queen Chicory might well have induced Princess Clematis to be born somewhat earlier than expected. She was a small baby and they often teased her that she had not been ready to come into the world, nor was she willing to be in it now, because she spent so much time day-dreaming and building castles in the air, that she might as well be living in the clouds!

Only today, King Vervain had found her designing a system of metal tubes which she planned to install throughout the castle so that she could talk down one end and the servants could hear her at the other. "Like a long hunting horn," the Princess had explained. "It would save the servants a lot of time if I could tell them what I wanted instead of them coming to my room for instructions."

King Vervain shuddered at the thought of elongated hunting horns snaking their way to every room of the castle, with voices blaring out of their ends. But, even as he told her to forget her impractical ideas, there was a feeling at the back of his mind that perhaps one day some of Princess Clematis' ideas might actually work.

My goodness, it was time for bed and he had not even started the list of guests for the party. How his mind had been wandering. As King Vervain roused himself, he did not see the Unicorn slip silently away. White Chestnut had been happily inserting all sorts of unwanted thoughts into King Vervain's mind. It was so easy to do and now he was off to find another victim to annoy. He did not have far to look.

Sitting at the table in her parlour, Mistress Olive was pondering the same problem as the king. She, too, knew that it was time to start planning Prince Walnut's birthday party. The happy co-incidence of his birthday falling at Hallow E'en gave King Vervain a fortunate excuse for giving a very large party to which he invited all the children from surrounding farms and villages. Many of the grown-ups joined in the fun, dressing up as fairies and witches, wizards and hobgoblins. King Vervain also wore fancy dress. It was the only day of the whole year when he did not have to wear his golden crown. There would be jugglers and acrobats, clowns and conjurers, minstrels and mummers, and it would be hard to tell who enjoyed the party more, the children or the grown ups.

Of all the King's children, Prince Walnut was Mistress Olive's favourite. When he was a baby, she had been his nurse. When he grew too big to need a nurse, King Vervain had made her Chief Housekeeper at the Castle. While very honoured, Mistress Olive found all the extra work very hard, overseeing all the cooks and gardeners, footmen and butlers, chamber maids and dressmakers. Right now, what Mistress Olive needed more than anything was a holiday, not another party to plan, but she loved Prince Walnut dearly and somehow she knew she would find the energy to get everything done.

She would ask Witch Hornbeam to help. Witch Hornbeam had taken charge of the Royal Nursery when Princess Clematis was born. Some thought she was too old for the job and certainly many wakeful nights had left her permanently tired, but, as the wife of Wizard Elm, and nearly as learned as he in the art of making medicines and potions, she had been the choice of King Vervain for the little princess. It was not thought that Princess Clematis would live, she was so tiny, but under Witch Hornbeam's loving care, she had grown up to be a beautiful young girl.

This year she had been crowned Queen of the May and, as

she danced around the May Pole, King Vervain had declared her the prettiest girl in his kingdom and no one had disagreed, except, of course, Princess Holly, who was immediately jealous and declared that she hated her sister, although no one else could understand what Princess Clematis had done to deserve it.

Mistress Olive went to the big castle kitchen where she found Witch Hornbeam fast asleep in front of the fire, with her cat sleeping at her feet. Poor Witch Hornbeam, her daily duties left her tired too. At times it was hard to know which of them was the more worn out, although Mistress Olive felt sure it must be her as she had so many more things to worry about.

Tonight she was more tired than usual and, much as she wanted to plan the party for her beloved Prince Walnut, somehow she could not concentrate. She would go to bed. After a good night's sleep she would feel better.

But sleep did not come. As Mistress Olive lay in the darkness, her mind was crowded with thoughts which would not let her rest. It was nearly dawn before she finally fell into a fitful slumber.

And we know why! White Chestnut had finally tired of his game and, as the first rays of sunlight lit up the top of the mountain, the mischievous little unicorn slipped back into his cave and settled himself down to sleep.

Chapter Six

In which a party is planned and the Troubadours come to town

Prince Walnut's birthday celebrations had been planned. After consulting Duke Vine, Mistress Olive, Witch Hornbeam, Wizard Elm and anybody else the King could think of who could be trusted to keep a secret, it had been decided to hold two events for Prince Walnut's birthday.

King Vervain had decided Prince Walnut was old enough to experience the excitement of a paperchase, which would take the prince and a small group of his special friends up hill and down dale, until they finally reached a secret destination where the two princesses, and a small group of their friends, would have been busy preparing a sumptuous birthday tea.

This event was to be a surprise for the prince, who would be expecting only the usual evening's entertainment. The arrangements for that could safely be left in the hands of the good and efficient Mistress Olive. Poor woman, how tired she looked! King Vervain promised himself that he would arrange for her to have a week off to visit her elderly mother, which he knew she wished to do. He would see to it immediately after the party — that is, if he could spare her, with the Christmas festivities so fast approaching.

A more difficult task was arranging the paper chase. Obviously, the best person to write the clues would be the school master, Mr. Gentian. Mr. Gentian was both pleased and honoured at being asked to arrange so important a function. Within an hour he had planned the cross country route over which the chase would pass, but the next task he found far harder. He needed to write the cryptic clues which would be hidden at each secret location along the way. He must not make them too easy, else they would be no fun. He must not make them too hard, or Prince Walnut and his friends might get lost and miss his birthday tea altogether.

In fact, Mr. Gentian found that, easy or difficult, it did not matter, he could think of no clues at all! Becoming disheartened, he set out to see his friend, Mr. Gorse.

Mr. Gorse was feeling depressed. Ever since he had retired from teaching, handing over the school into the capable hands of Mr. Gentian, he had felt he had nothing to live for. Every day seemed as pointless as the day before. He tried to put on a brave face so that the people of Merry Hi Hi would not know how 'down' he felt. When Mr. Gentian arrived to tell him of his problem, Mr. Gorse felt grumpy. He said a paperchase so late in the year was a silly idea because the weather would be too cold and it would probably rain. Declaring that it was a waste of time inventing any clues because the valley would probably be covered in fog and no one able to read them, Mr. Gorse settled down to the task in hand with what might almost seem to be enthusiasm. He would not admit it, but he thoroughly enjoyed inventing cryptic clues, which he unashamedly hoped would be too hard. If the prince and his friends got lost on the moors, well, it would be no more than he had forecast!

With the arrangements for the festivities well in hand, King Vervain was able to turn his attention to his favourite part of the day — the entertainment! Travelling troubadours always came to town for Hallow E'en and he was looking forward to watching the acrobats and jugglers. It was the juggler, Impatiens, who fascinated him most. While acrobats needed to be born with supple bodies (which King Vervain knew, most decidedly, he had not!), it would seem that anybody could learn to juggle, provided they had two hands and lots of concentration.

Each year King Vervain watched in awe as Impatiens juggled more and more balls in the air. Most incredible of all was when Impatiens walked a tightrope across the Great Dining Hall while juggling at the same time. While the acrobats worked together, Impatiens preferred to work on his own. "If something goes wrong, then there is no one to blame but me," he would say.

Each year King Vervain vowed to himself that he would learn to juggle. He did not want anyone to laugh at his efforts, but taking his dogs for a walk gave him a good excuse to carry several balls. When well out of sight, he would try to juggle as Impatiens did, but he was lucky if he could keep two balls in the air, let alone ten!

Besides Impatiens, there would be Brother Pine, the minstrel. Brother Pine would stay at the castle until Christmas, which greatly pleased the king because he had never heard anyone with such a beautiful voice and he loved to hear him sing the Christmas songs. The other troubadours would travel to the neighbouring kingdom, which had once been Brother Pine's home. Brother Pine would not go with them. He felt so guilty because he had failed to save one of his friends from drowning, although he had done his best, that he could not return to face his friends and family. "I should never have let him go swimming alone," he would say. "It is my fault that he died." Nothing anyone could say could help him to forgive himself. "I forgive the sins of others," he replied. "That is easy to do. But to forgive myself? That is the hardest thing of all."

While King Vervain was sorry that Brother Pine still felt so guilty, even after all these years, he knew it was an ill wind that blew nobody any good, and the Brother's beautiful voice would lead the singing of the carols at the castle Christmas morn. King Vervain could hear Brother Pine practicing now. The song seemed beautiful, but, no matter how well Brother Pine sang, he always believed he could, and should, do better.

The troubadours brought with them news of happenings in far off countries and stories of things unheard of in the kingdom of Merry Hi Hi. Willow, the leader of the mummers, said there were countries across the sea where it was warm all the year round, no frost or snow! He told of mountains which were on fire inside and which spat out red hot ash when the spirits were angry. Much to his disappointment, Willow had never actually seen this occur. It always happened when he was not there! "It's not fair," Willow moaned. "I always seem to miss out."

Now Willow was complaining again. King Vervain had written a play for the party and given the main part to Prince Walnut. Willow felt that, as principle actor, he should have been given the leading part. To make matters worse, Willow had been woken at the crack of dawn by the clattering of horses' hooves as King Vervain and his men rode over the drawbridge for their early morning ride. He complained to everyone at the castle who was willing to listen. No wonder his friends called him Whingy Willow!

A more popular member of the troupe was Cerato, the soothsayer. Some people called her "silver tongued" because she always foretold things which were pleasing to those who paid to have their fortunes told. Her counsel was a little vague at times, but that did not stop others from constantly seeking her advice, however misguided it might later turn out to be.

Soothsayer Cerato was a cousin of Wizard Elm and even he was glad to have the opportunity to unburden some of his responsibilities during her stay. She told him that Gnome Chestnut Bud's infatuation with Water Violet was passing and that next year, when the ice on the lake melted, he would not be resuming his swim to the lily pad. Wizard Elm was very glad to hear this, as Chestnut Bud's continuing cough was causing some concern.

Everybody else in the valley seemed to be over their coughs and colds, which was a great relief, because Wizard Elm was in charge of the fancy dress costumes for the Hallow E'en party. He and his wife, Witch Hornbeam, had looked out all the costumes that had been worn last year and were busy mending them.

King Vervain always wanted to go as a wizard and borrowed Wizard Elm's spare cloak for the occasion. Considering King Vervain's expanding waistline, Wizard Elm was glad the king's costume was a loose fitting cloak!

Witch Hornbeam had been put in charge of baking The Cake. King Vervain was hoping that Witch Hornbeam would go down to the lake to speak to Mistress Heather, who was believed to have added another ingredient to her famous cake recipe. She might be persuaded to part with her secret, especially as it was known that the gnome people were afraid of witches and she would not want to make Witch Hornbeam angry.

King Vervain could smell the cake cooking. Yes! He felt sure that Witch Hornbeam had obtained the secret recipe. He was sure he had never smelt a cake as good before.

Princess Clematis was helping, although Witch Hornbeam called it hindering. At last the cake was in the oven and Princess Clematis was seated at the table, with instructions to call Witch Hornbeam when all the sand had run through the hour glass.

While Princess Clematis was dreamily staring into the fire, it suddenly occurred to her that it might help the fisherman to catch more fish if she could design a boat with a lid on it, which could go under the water to find the fish. She was pondering the problem of how the fishermen would see, when she became aware of the very angry Witch Hornbeam taking a very burnt cake out of the oven.

"You might as well feed this to the chickens," cried Witch Hornbeam. "It is good for nothing else." Princess Clematis took the burnt cake and hurried down to the chicken shed. "At least the chickens are not fussy," she thought to herself. "They do not mind their food being hard and dry. Perhaps we could bake them some dry food which would feed them in the winter when the yard is covered in frost and snow."

She was so delighted with this idea that she ran back to tell Witch Hornbeam, quite forgetting to collect the fresh eggs which Witch Hornbeam needed to bake another cake.

Chapter Seven

In which Lady Beech is puzzled and Red Chestnut is worried

Lady Beech, Sir Scleranthus' mother, had offered to help Mistress Olive with preparations for the party. Lady Beech was renowned throughout the kingdom for her beautiful needlework. Her artistic talent, combined with her fine eye for detail, enabled her to make the most exquisite altar cloths and banners for the church and castle. She worked on them every day with as much dedication and effort as her son gave to his efforts to improve his physical prowess.

But it was not for her sewing abilities that Lady Beech was welcomed at this time. Her keen eye for detail extended to all areas of life. She demanded the same dedication and perfection from her servants in the performance of their work as she gave to hers. Woe betide them if an ornament was out of place or a picture hung crookedly on the wall. And woe betide her housekeeper if all the accounts were not correctly kept. Every evening when it grew too dark to continue her needlework, she sent for the housekeeper to bring her the day's accounts and, by candlelight, she carefully studied the record of every item that had been purchased.

It was her intention to make sure, not only that nothing was overlooked which needed to be purchased for the party, but that everything was bought at the very best price. "King Vervain is too generous," she would say. "If no one else checked the bills, the villagers would charge him far too much and he would pay without giving it a thought."

And Lady Beech was right. King Vervain enjoyed planning big events, but the little details, such as how much they cost, he rarely bothered about.

Lady Beech had made a list of all the items she considered needed to be purchased for the party. She handed it to her maid, Aspen, with instructions for it to be taken at once to Mistress Olive, before she went to bed. As Aspen hurried across the castle battlements, a gust of wind blew the list out of her hand and, in dismay, she watched it float away over the castle wall and out of sight.

What would Lady Beech say? Aspen trembled at the thought. She did not know that the bad fairy, Mimulus, had caused the gust of wind to snatch the paper out of her hand. When mortals are in a state of excitement, it is easy for the bad fairies to cause mischief. The unicorn, White Chestnut, joined Mimulus hovering around the maid that night, filling her mind with anxious thoughts of what Lady Beech would say in the morning, causing the poor girl to shake with fear.

Unknown to her, kindly dragon Red Chestnut, saw what happened as he gazed down upon the village from his mountain cave. He was full of concern for little Aspen and winged his way down to the castle walls where the errant list was caught in the branch of a bush. Very gently he blew a little hot air from his nostrils, being very careful not to singe or burn the paper.

Gradually it came loose and Red Chestnut put all his skills into practice as he gently blew the paper round the side of the castle and guided it so that it wafted up to the window of the chamber where Lady Beech lay soundly sleeping. In fluttered the paper, coming to rest at the foot of Lady Beech's bed, where she found it when she woke the next morning.

"How strange," she thought. "I was sure I had given this list to the maid last night. I must be getting forgetful!" She rang the bell to summon Aspen, who entered the room in such a state of fright at the scolding she was expecting to receive, that her knees shook like jelly, her hands trembled, her teeth chattered, and her face was as white as a ghost's.

"Good gracious me, girl!" exclaimed Lady Beech. "You must be ill. Go back to bed at once. I was going to ask you to take this list to Mistress Olive, but I will do it myself."

Aspen never did know what had happened, but she enjoyed her day in bed, especially as Lady Beech (who was really very kind) arranged for the best chicken soup to be sent up for her lunch, together with hot bread rolls, straight from the oven, spread with freshly churned butter!

Duke Vine's mother, the Dowager Duchess Crab Apple, was most disturbed to hear that one of the maids was ill. She immediately suspected that the child had the plague and persuaded Lady Beech that Aspen should not return to her duties for at least a week.

If Lady Beech was fussy about details, the Dowager Duchess Crab Apple was fussy about dirt and germs! She believed sickness lurked everywhere and her servants were forever scrubbing and polishing, not because that made her castle look good (which is what would have concerned Lady Beech) but because she was determined that nothing unhealthy would find its way into her fortress.

The Dowager Duchess Crab Apple was as fussy about her personal cleanliness as she was about the cleanliness of her rooms. Every evening her servants carried buckets of hot water up the stairs to her chamber so that she could bathe in front of the fire. "Cleanliness is next to Godliness," she would say.

Each morning she stood in front of her mirror and studied her face very carefully, in case some spot or blemish had appeared in the night. If Wizard Elm and Witch Hornbeam were skilled at making potions to help sick folk get well, the Dowager Duchess was equally skilled at making potions for beautifying the skin and hair.

Princess Holly used to consider her an old fuss pot but, a young lady herself now, Princess Holly had taken to seeking out the Dowager Duchess' company, to discuss the relative merits of egg white or honey as a face mask and chamomile or sage as a rinse for the hair. And as for diet! Nobody knew more than the Dowager Duchess Crab Apple about which foods should be eaten to keep the figure trim and to help nails grow long and strong.

Now, while all this activity was going on in the castle, the bad fairies were hard at work, too! Mimulus was busy making all the children nervous at the thought of being invited to a party at the castle. She was giving the mummers attacks of stage fright at the prospect of performing the play which King Vervain had written especially for the occasion.

Rock Rose knew that Prince Walnut did not like thunderstorms, so she was making preparations with the North Wind for a truly humungous storm to break while he was on the paperchase and Cherry Plum was turning her attention to the home of the Court Jester, Agrimony. Although Agrimony put on a happy face when entertaining the king at the castle, behind his smile there lay a heavy heart. His wife, Sweet Chestnut, was crippled from a fall she had had some years before and had difficulty moving about their cottage at all. Agrimony was able to be home much of the day to help his long suffering wife, but in the evenings he had to leave her alone while he told jokes at the castle and exchanged riddles with the king.

Queen Chicory had arranged for Sweet Chestnut to be brought to the castle to share in the Hallow E'en festivities. Now Cherry Plum was planning to make her pains so bad that evening that she would not be able to get in the carriage to go to the party. "She will have to sit at home all alone and in pain, while everybody else is enjoying themselves," gloated Cherry Plum. "That should push her to the limit of her endurance."

With everybody else doing all the work and worrying, King Vervain was free to hustle about his castle with great enthusiasm, satisfying himself that this was going to be the biggest and best Hallow E'en party ever. He understood how long a day can seem to children when they are waiting for a treat in the evening, so he arranged for Wild Oat, the blacksmith's son, to organize entertainment for the children during the day.

Wild Oat was as energetic as his sister, Wild Rose, was lazy. The only problem was that he never persevered with anything for long, so he never achieved anything worthwhile. He could have been better than Sir Scleranthus at jousting but became bored with the daily practice and decided to take up falconry instead. Once he had trained the falcon, he became bored with that and gave the falcon to Larch to care for. Larch was quite overwhelmed at the thought of caring for such a precious bird, but Wild Oat said "Rubbish. You can do it" — and to his surprise Larch found that he could!

King Vervain wondered what Wild Oat's latest interest would be. He glanced out of the castle window and saw Wild Oat in the courtyard with Impatiens, who was teaching him to juggle. Already he was able to keep four balls in the air. King Vervain scowled! But he would not let his jealousy spoil his day for long. "He has many talents. Maybe Soothsayer Cerato will know what he should do. I must ask her before she leaves."

And so, in the valley below and in the mountains above, each was busy with their plans, while the gentle dragon, Red Chestnut, watched and worried.

Chapter Eight

In which some plans go well, others do not and everyone grows a little wiser

Hallow E'en had come and gone. The party had been a great success, although the paperchase had been the cause of a few anxious moments.

Mr. Gentian and Mr. Gorse had made the course quite hard. Prince Walnut and his friends found deciphering the clues very tricky. Some were straightforward, but others really stretched their brains. They had started out early in the morning and it was nearly dark by the time the exhausted party had reached the secret destination where their party awaited them.

The day had started out clear and sunny, but in the afternoon an unexpected storm suddenly blew up. Prince Walnut was already becoming tired and insisted that one of the clues was to lead them down the hill to a small waterfall when, in fact, it was to lead them up the hill to the large waterfall. When the Prince finally admitted he was wrong, they had twice as far to climb back up the mountain to the Great Falls. It was here the storm had come rolling in and the bedraggled party clambered over the slippery rocks behind the Falls into the safe refuge of the caves behind.

"It's strange how I always thought the Falls so fierce and scary. I used to feel as though their thunderous waters wished to dash me to pieces on the rocks below," Prince Walnut recalled, "but with the storm outside, I felt quite safe within. The roar of the waters drowned out the noise of the storm and I felt their strength as a protection, not a threat."

"I agree," said Sir Scleranthus. "There seemed to be a great peace among the moving water. I wondered how anything so moving could bring such a sense of peace."

"Ever changing, never changing eternity," mused Princess Clematis.

"I was so tired and thirsty," Prince Walnut continued, "but after drinking water which had collected among the rocks, I seemed to find new strength and courage. I understand why Wizard Elm goes there so often. He carries some of the Rock Water home with him because he says is brings him strength."

"It turned out to be a good thing that you led us on that wild goose chase down the hill," said Larch, "otherwise we would already have left the safety of the Great Falls and been in the open meadow when the storm struck." Little did he know that that had been Rock Rose's plan! It was Red Chestnut and White Chestnut who made sure her plan did not work.

Now, I know you will be surprised to hear that White Chestnut actually did something helpful for a change, but White Chestnut was feeling cross with Rock Rose at the time. How was he to know that the previous Wednesday she had been planning to terrify everyone at the castle by causing a fire while they were all asleep? White Chestnut had chosen that very night to keep Duke Vine awake with lots of silly, worrying thoughts.

Duke Vine, going down to the kitchen to fetch a cup of hot milk, had discovered the fire which was already burning fiercely. He had bellowed so loudly into the metal tubes which Princess Clematis had persuaded Mr. Oak to install in the servants' quarters, that no one in the castle was left in any doubt as to their effectiveness!

Within minutes, servants arrived from everywhere with buckets of water and brooms to beat out the flames. Thanks to Duke Vine's quick thinking, no one had been hurt.

Rock Rose had been so angered by the spoiling of her plan that she had forbidden White Chestnut to leave the cave at night for a whole week. White Chestnut thought this most unfair and was happy to help Red Chestnut spoil yet another of Rock Rose's plans.

And so White Chestnut had put the thought into Prince Walnut's head to go down the mountain instead of up. The delay ensured that the party was not out in the open when the storm hit. It was fortunate for White Chestnut that Rock Rose did not realize what had happened.

Cherry Plum's wicked plan had fared no better. Wizard Elm had visited the cottage of Agrimony the afternoon of the paper chase and had felt the presence of Cherry Plum as she tried to torment poor, long suffering Sweet Chestnut. While Agrimony was helping Sweet Chestnut to butter the hot scones for tea, Wizard Elm took the opportunity to recite one of his most powerful protective spells and Cherry Plum had been quite unable to enter the house.

"That was quite a day," recalled Wild Oat. "While all of you were sheltering from the storm in the cave, I was looking after the children. Some of them were frightened but on the whole they were very good. I played games with them so they would forget about the storm and I enjoyed the day so much that I have decided to become a teacher. I will be helping Mr. Gentian with the village school. For the first time in my life, I feel that I have found something really worthwhile at which to work."

King Vervain smiled to himself. Soothsayer Cerato had told him that Wild Oat would soon work out for himself his path, which would bring much reward to him and benefit the village.

Much as he enjoyed Hallow E'en, King Vervain enjoyed this evening more, for it was Christmas Eve. For days now preparations for Christmas had been in full swing and the castle was gaily festooned with decorations which everybody had helped to make. Each year the castle looked more festive than the year before. Even lackadaisical Wild Rose had roused herself to help and her smile of pride as she watched her paper-chain being hung in its place in the Great Hall gave King Vervain hope that she might start to make more effort in the year to come.

Now a hush was falling over the castle as the servants were retiring to their quarters. King Vervain was sitting in front of a large fire in the old nursery, where he always spent Christmas Eve with the Prince and Princesses and some of their closest friends.

Outside the snow had been falling, but inside the castle it was warm and cosy. Darkness had fallen and the flickering candles cast a cheerful glow around the room. The Christmas tree had been decorated and the Star of Bethlehem had been placed at the top. It was a beautiful star, which Mr. Oak had made out of gold and silver. It glittered and shone in the light of the fire.

"Christmas seems to start when we place our Star of Bethlehem on the tree," mused Princess Holly. "It seems to bring its own special peace. Somehow, when I look at it, all the hurts and unhappiness of the year seem to fade. I wish it could shine for ever."

"The stars shine every night. It's just that some nights the clouds are between us and them and we do not see their light. I am sure the Star of Bethlehem is shining all the time, if we could but see it."

Princess Holly glanced across at her sister. How like Princess Clematis to say something like that. In the warm glow of the fire light, Princess Holly saw that she was, indeed, as pretty as her father had said and, as she gazed once more at the star shining on the tree, she felt her jealousy melt away.

Princess Holly looked across the room to where Sweet Chestnut was sitting next to her husband, Agrimony. She wondered if Sweet Chestnut, too, felt the comfort of the star? She hoped so, for Sweet Chestnut had suffered more than anyone else. Princess Holly felt ashamed. "How silly I was to be jealous of something so trivial, when I have so much to be thankful for," she said to herself. She resolved that next year she would be better.

Gnome Chestnut Bud was also resolving to be better next year. He was sitting on the edge of the lake, staring up at the stars twinkling in the heavens. How bright they looked on this crystal clear night. Tomorrow the Christmas festivities would begin. He surveyed his waistcoat thoughtfully. The button Mrs. Heather had sewn back into place was still there. He hoped it would last through Christmas dinner! Next week would be New Year. He would start his diet then, really he would.

He glanced across the lake and saw nymph Water Violet skating across the frozen surface. How graceful she looked. He wished he could join her, but he knew that she was happy with her own company, so he resisted the temptation.

Wizard Elm, being wise, was busy in his cellar, making lots and lots of indigestion mix!

Each person was thinking over the year that had passed.

"It's strange," said Prince Walnut to his father, "but while we were on the paperchase, all I could think of was how far there was to go, how difficult the clues were and how cold and hungry I was. I was so grateful for those parts of the chase which were over flat ground. But now, it is the difficult parts I most enjoy recalling."

"That is because you put in effort," said King Vervain. "One only grows through effort, whether physically, mentally, emotionally or spiritually. I am sure it was solving the hardest clues which gave you the most pleasure."

"Of course," replied Prince Walnut. "And the party tea was such a lovely surprise. What strange creatures we humans are, that we need life to be made difficult for it to be made interesting — even if we do not think it much fun at the time!"

King Vervain smiled. "Remember. Life is Godde's paperchase, my son."

The Pilgrim's Hymn

He who would true valour see,
Let him come hither;
Here one will constant be,
Come wind, come weather.
There's no discouragement
Will make him once relent
His first avowed intent
To be a pilgrim

John Bunyan

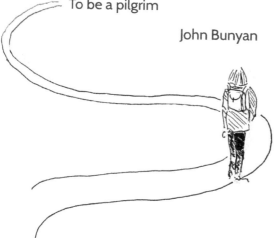

About the Author

Born in London, Denise Carrington-Smith came to Australia in 1967, raising her family in Melbourne, where she lived for nearly thirty years. During this time, Denise took up the study and practice of yoga, which she taught for a number of years.

It was through yoga that Denise became interested in healing, training first as a natural therapist and homœopath and then as a psychologist and clinical hypnotherapist.

For some years, Denise lectured in herbalism, the Bach Flower Remedies and homœopathy before becoming Principal of the Victorian College of Classical Homœopathy. She also served as President of the Australian Federation of Homœopaths. During this time, Denise continued to offer regular workshops for practitioners and others interested in the study of the Bach Flower Remedies.

In 1995, she retired to Far North Queensland, returning to University where she took up the study of archæology, specializing in the study of evolutionary theory, which was the subject of her doctoral thesis.

Denise has seven children, seventeen grandchildren and four great-grandchildren (so far).

www.ingramcontent.com/pod-product-compliance
Lightning Source LLC
LaVergne TN
LVHW022201240125
801994LV00046B/1259